The Kinder, Gentler Cancer Treatment

Insulin Potentiation Targeted LowDose™ Therapy

Targeting the Cancer Cells
          ...Not the Patient!

The Best Answer for Cancer Foundation[SM]

Thriving While Surviving[SM]

Contributing Physicians

Steven G. Ayre, MD
Hendrieka Fitzpatrick, MD
David C. Korn, DDS, DO, MD (H)
Constantine A. Kotsanis, MD
Richard Linchitz, MD
Thomas Lodi, MD
Frank Shallenberger, MD, HMD

Contributing Cancer Survivors

Annie Brandt
Charles Gray
Richard Linchitz, MD
Michael Short

The Kinder, Gentler Cancer Treatment

Insulin Potentiation Targeted LowDose™ Therapy

Targeting the Cancer Cells
...Not the Patient!

Table of Contents

What is The Best Answer for Cancer Foundation℠ And What Do We Mean by "The Best Answer for Cancer"?

We are a small group of cancer survivors, laypeople, and concerned physicians supporting Insulin Potentiation Targeted LowDose™ Therapy (IPTLD™) – Kinder, gentler chemotherapy...

WHAT DO WE MEAN BY A KINDER, GENTLER CHEMOTHERAPY?

Most people hear chemotherapy and react with fear. Did you know that 40 percent of chemotherapy patients reported side effects as their biggest concern compared to 32 percent who thought surviving cancer was their biggest concern?** That is because we have all seen friends, relatives, or just John Q. Public devastated by the effects of their chemotherapy.

IPTLD™ offers the patient the ability to have the power of the chemo directed only to his or her cancer cells, not the patient's entire body. This approach eliminates or significantly reduces the dreaded side effects of conventional chemo.

WHAT DO WE MEAN BY "THE BEST ANSWER FOR CANCER"?

We believe The "Best" Answer for Cancer is our philosophy here at The Best Answer for Cancer Foundation℠:

- A solid holistic and integrated platform of healing and strengthening components (mind/body, spirituality, diet/nutrition, detox, immune system boosting, and exercise) that support and strengthen the patient's body to further increase the effectiveness of...

- A targeted cancer therapy that destroys the cancer, not the patient.

The Best Answer for Cancer Foundation℠ funds education and research to support IPTLD™, a kinder, gentler chemotherapy. You can help...

Your oncologist will strongly advise chemotherapy to kill cancer. The standard approach is to give you as much chemotherapy as your body can tolerate...in THE HOPE...that the chemo will kill the cancer before the drugs kill you.

IPTLD™* is a kinder, gentler way to fight cancer with chemotherapy drugs that are approved by the FDA (Federal Drug Administration). While searching for a way to selectively deliver drugs to diseased cells only, Dr. Donato Perez Garcia I discovered this treatment in 1929. His development of the therapy led him to try it on cancer in 1946, with great success. With this approach, your immune system and vital body organs stay working and you have almost no side effects. This means you should not lose your hair, you should not be nauseous, and your blood counts should stay normal...generally speaking, you feel great.

Patients report that IPTLD™ chemotherapy gives them the same or better results than those of conventional chemotherapy...beating cancer while living life fully...Thriving While Surviving℠!

An important goal of The Best Answer for Cancer Foundation℠ is to put IPTLD™ through clinical trials in order to have it accepted as a "standard of care." Even though IPTLD™ has been used successfully on cancer since 1946, the pharmaceutical companies have never performed a clinical trial. Therefore, it is still considered an off-label use of insulin and chemotherapy drugs and, as such, is not yet a standard offering in your oncologist's office. Having gone through IPT myself for advanced-stage metastatic breast cancer, I want this option for every cancer patient in the world!

Do you know that, in 2005, the American Cancer Society published mortality data*** that showed that from 1950 to 2002, the mortality rate had dropped significantly for all major chronic diseases **except cancer? The mortality rate of cancer remained the same!** The significance of this cannot be overlooked.

The use of IPTLD™ needs more research as well as clinical trials mentioned previously. While pharmaceutical companies are spending billions of dollars on research into new drugs, they could be easily testing the effectiveness of existing drugs with the IPTLD™ therapy. In essence, this would give patients another option: the option of a targeted therapy using the power of existing, proven chemotherapy drugs. It would give patients the choice of a kinder, gentler—yet effective—therapy for cancer.

The pharmaceutical companies, when approached about clinical trials, replied that they had already tested all the drugs involved and could not see the financial value of testing a therapy that used lower doses of the drugs.

Currently, insurance carriers do not normally cover IPT/IPTLD™ treatments, even though the therapy uses FDA-approved drugs. We are encouraging patients to write to their insurance companies, the media, their federal representatives, and senators to encourage acceptance of this successful off-label usage of FDA-approved drugs.

Your contribution to The Best Answer for Cancer Foundation[SM] will add to this important work. Help us give every cancer patient the additional choice to do this therapy, and to experience Thriving While Surviving[SM] cancer!

*The name IPT (Insulin Potentiation Therapy) has recently been changed to IPTLD™ (Insulin Potentiation Targeted LowDose™). **IPTLD™** is the current name (researched, reserved, and assigned in 2006 by Annie Brandt and the board of The Best Answer for Cancer Foundation[SM] to more accurately describe the therapy) for that same procedure. Only the name has changed to better represent the technique; the therapy remains the same. Throughout this book, you will see both names. Please consider them synonymous.

**Source: www.bymyside.com/pdf/InfectionBackgrounder.pdf (Roper Starch survey)

*** Sources: http://www.cdc.gov/nchs/deaths.htm, 1950 Mortality Data – CDC/NCHS, NVSS and Mortality Revised.

❀

Dedication and Acknowledgements
The Best Answer for Cancer Foundation^{SM}

Thriving While Surviving^{SM}

By Annie Brandt, Executive Director

Annie Brandt is the Cofounder, along with Rachel Best, of The Best Answer for Cancer Foundation^{SM}, established in 2004 as a *project* of another 501(c)(3). Annie and Rachel found they both had cancer in common and they decided that they were not going to use conventional treatment since they had a mutual desire to maintain a high quality of life while killing the cancer. Rachel had a recurrence of ovarian cancer and Annie had advanced-stage metastatic breast cancer. According to the conventional doctors, neither one of them had a good prognosis.

After experiencing the benefits of IPT, they decided they had to tell the world about IPT/IPTLD™ and put their efforts into bringing this option to cancer patients everywhere.

In 2006, Rachel passed away of an infection entirely unrelated to her cancer. Annie then took action to legitimize the foundation as a formal 501(c)(3), and is the Founder and Executive Director of The Best Answer for Cancer Foundation^{SM}. annie@ElkaBest.org

This book is dedicated primarily to cancer patients everywhere, and any person who is interested in *Thriving <u>While</u> Surviving*^{SM}, as well as God from Whom all blessings flow. The former inspires and fires me; the latter always loves and supports me.

Additionally, there must be accolades and recognition given to Dr. Donato Perez Garcia I and his descendants. To Dr. Donato Perez Garcia I for discovering and pioneering the therapy of IPT in 1929, and for being curious enough to see its effects on other diseases to try it on cancer in 1942. To Dr. Donato Perez Garcia II for further exploring its applications for cancer and chronic diseases. Finally, to Dr. Donato Perez Garcia III for bringing IPT to the world, with the invaluable assistance and support of Dr. Steven G. Ayre. Dr. Donato III and Dr. Steven Ayre are true pioneers: traveling the world to train new physicians; writing white papers and giving seminars on the value of IPT; forging relationships with key government and medical bodies such as the National Cancer Institute's Office of Cancer Complementary and Alternative Medicine. Dr. Donato III was my IPT physician, and I credit him largely with my survival. You can read more about him in my story later in this book.

Without these four men, I would not have found IPT, and I would most likely not be alive today.

The IPTLD™ physicians who contributed to this book are due our sincere thanks for their continuous support of us at The Best Answer for Cancer Foundation^{SM}. They are just a few of the brilliant, dedicated, and compassionate physicians that offer IPT/IPTLD™. Additional heartfelt thanks are due to all of the IPTLD™ physicians worldwide who have joined in our effort to collaborate, communicate, and cooperate in order to increase the awareness of IPT/IPTLD™ around the world. You can read more about them, or find more IPTLD™ physicians, at www.IPTforcancer.com or www.IPTLD.com.

There are over three hundred trained IPTLD™ physicians in the world. Through the efforts of the staff of The Best Answer for Cancer Foundation^{SM} and our wonderful volunteers, we have located over forty of these physicians. The Best Answer for Cancer Foundation^{SM} Medical Advisory Board and the Board of Directors have certified these forty physicians. The two boards have worked together to establish standards in training and in the delivery of the IPTLD™ therapy that resulted in IPTLD™ certification. Our goal is to locate and bring more physicians on board to offer this kind and gentle—yet very effective—therapy to patients all over the world. If you are an IPT physician and would like to join our Foundation Board-certified organization of physicians, or you are a physician that is interested in learning IPTLD™, please contact Rebecca Ayre at rebecca@iptforcancer.com or call us at 512-342-8181 or 630-321-9010.

Last, but certainly not least in the level of acknowledgement, I would like to thank the staff and volunteers of The Best Answer for Cancer Foundation^{SM}. Special love and gratitude go to my two volunteer directors, Rebecca Ayre and LaMae Weber, who accepted titles in lieu of pay and who have been my strong and cheerful cohorts as we have gone through the growth process. The Foundation would not be where it is today without these two women, who not only bring great ideas to the table, but also stimulate, support, and keep me sane and laughing at the same time—a great combination for creativity!

To our new volunteers, Rosalind Joseph, Connie Gonzales, and Lindsey Mewbourn, thank you for your enthusiasm, energy, and efficiency!

To all of our doctors' support staff, know that your "behind the scenes" efforts and dedication are indeed appreciated and recognized:

Nicole Snyder, Lindsay Moore, Jana Miller, Shena Korn, Kristine Hanafi, Rita Linchitz, Judy Shallenberger, Clothilde Canale, and Tracey Emmons, to name just a few.

Sincere thanks to Dr. Les Breitman and Dr. Steven Ayre, fellow Board of Directors members and experienced IPTLD™ physicians, who help educate and support us in our efforts with IPTLD™. To Rachel Best, of blessed memory, who lives on with us in our work, and Bill Harvey who helped energize and organize us. Finally, to Beverly Kotsanis and Marge Woodard, without whom we could not have published this book, I direct the praise and gratitude of all who enjoy this book.

Annie Brandt
annie@ElkaBest.org

Disclaimer*

The information presented in this book is based on the experiences of the authors and contributors. It is intended for informational and educational purposes only. **In no way should this book be used as a substitute for your own physician's advice.**

Because medicine and particularly oncology (the medical field that specializes in cancer and cancer therapy) is an ever-changing science, readers are encouraged to confirm the information contained herein with other sources, including their own personal oncologists (doctors who specialize in cancer.) The authors of this book have used sources they believe to be reliable to substantiate the information provided. However, because of the possibility of human error or changes in medical sciences, neither the authors, publisher, editors, nor any other party who has been involved in the preparation or publication of this work warrants that the information contained herein is in every respect accurate or complete. They are not responsible for any errors or omissions or for the results obtained from the use of such information. This is especially true when a person with cancer receives Insulin Potentiation Targeted LowDose™ Therapy (aka Insulin Potentiation Therapy) or any of the therapies described in this book and a bad result occurs. The authors, publisher, and editors of this book do not warrant that Insulin Potentiation Targeted LowDose™ or any of the therapies described in this book will be effective in treating any medical condition, including cancer, and cannot guarantee or endorse any type of cancer therapy or practitioner who treats cancer patients.

No major therapy is 100 percent effective. This includes surgery, radiation, chemotherapy (with or without Insulin Potentiation Targeted LowDose™), or any other therapies described in this book, including alternative therapies. Thus, this book guarantees no particular results for the cancer patient or any other person reading it.

It is the responsibility of the individual cancer patient to thoroughly research the various cancer treatment options and discuss these options with their families, friends, and other confidants, as well as their health care providers, including their oncologists, before deciding on a particular treatment course. If the consensus is that Insulin Potentiation Therapy is to be given, it is still up to the individual cancer patient and the above individuals to choose a physician who is competent in the particular treatment modality. **As of yet, there is no American Medical Association (AMA) board certification available in Insulin Potentiation Targeted LowDose™ to ensure competency in this treatment. The Board of Directors and the Medical Advisory Board of The Best Answer for Cancer Foundation℠ provide certification concerned with the verification of practitioner medical credentials, procedures, training, and the issuance of continuing medical education credits.** Any licensed medical or osteopathic doctor in the United States can perform Insulin Potentiation Targeted LowDose™ according to the law. To see a directory of The IPT/IPTLD™ Physicians certified by The Best Answer for Cancer Foundation℠ Board of Directors and Medical Advisory Board, go to Appendix B in this book or www. iptforcancer.com/ipt/search.php. All certified physicians have completed a training course with an IPTLD™ Instructor and their AMA board-certified credentials have been verified.

Physicians should use and apply Insulin Potentiation Targeted LowDose™ and the other therapies described in this book only after they have received extensive training and demonstrated the ability to administer the treatment safely. The authors, publisher, editors, and any other persons involved in this work are not responsible if physicians who are unqualified in the use of Insulin Potentiation Targeted LowDose™ (a) administer the treatment based solely on the contents of this book or (b) receive training but do not administer it safely and a bad result occurs.

If Insulin Potentiation Targeted LowDose™ or any other treatment regime described in this book appears to apply to your condition, the authors, publisher, and editors recommend that a formal evaluation be performed by a physician who is competent in treating cancer patients with these various treatments. Those desiring Insulin Potentiation Targeted LowDose™ or any other treatment modality described in this book should make medical decisions with the aid of a personal physician. No medical decisions should be made solely on the contents or recommendations made in this book.

The people in this book are real. Their stories are true. Some of their names, identifying characteristics, and facts have been altered to protect their privacy.

*Source: *Used with permission of Hauser, R., and Hauser, M., Treating Cancer with Insulin Potentiation Therapy, 2002. Oak Park, IL. Beulah Land Press.*

INTRODUCTION

CANCER and Me and IPT

By Steven G. Ayre, M.D.

A leader and pioneer of IPT therapy in the United States, Steven G. Ayre was the first American physician trained in IPT/IPTLD™ and the first American physician to bring this therapy to the United States. Dr. Ayre trained with Dr. Perez Garcia y Bellon in 1976 and again with Dr. Perez Garcia in 1997. He has been instrumental in providing the scientific rationale for the treatment and is a certified instructor of IPTLD™.

Dr. Ayre is the Medical Director of Contemporary Medicine in Burr Ridge, Illinois. He has thirty years of experience with "Integrative Medicine."

Conditions treated with IPT: Dr. Ayre uses IPT to treat cancer.
Practice Focus: Offers comprehensive cancer care (IPT, Nutritional Biochemistry, and Mind/Body Medicine) with a kinder and gentler approach.

Contact:	**Steven G. Ayre, MD and Ather A. Malik, DO**
	Contemporary Medicine
Address:	322 Burr Ridge Pkwy
	Burr Ridge, IL 60527
Phone:	630-321-9010
Fax:	630-321-9018
Web site:	www.contemporarymedicine.net
E-mail:	info@contemporarymedicine.net

Back in 1975, I was a young doctor busy with the practice of general medicine in my hometown of Montreal. I was keenly interested in the burgeoning of alternative medicine going on at that time—megavitamin therapies, nutrition, herbs and the like. I was also particularly focused on the alternative methods for treating cancer. Families touched by cancer's curse would congregate in my office, distraught, frightened, and yet hopeful for The Miracle. With each new addition to the list of "good stuff for cancer" hopes would rise, and then they would fall... Apart from a measure of emotional comfort, the truth is that I could offer them little of substance. I found myself facing an entirely new situation. All around there was a tremendous need for help, and so little in the way of useful resources.

One day in my office—it was right after lunch on a hot and sultry July afternoon—I had a consultation with one of these cancer patients and the patient's family. The patients always had that particularly pained kind of look, face highlighted by a brownish hue. Chemotherapy. I recognized they gave it their best shot just by being there. I went through my usual steps: this dietary advice or that new supplement, and another go-round with some new self-help hint or yoga posture. Right after this family left the office area, the very next chart I picked up from the chart holder was yet another of these desperate families with cancer. At that moment, I felt I just couldn't face it. I turned back into my office, and closed the door. Then I got down on my knees and I prayed to God—for something to help these wretched people. Anything.

Please...

And then—magnificently—this, my prayer, was answered! Unaccustomed as I am to establishing contact with Higher Beings, I am certain that I did indeed experience this. And furthermore, over the ensuing weeks, through various and sundry avenues, I got literally rained upon by numerous alternative cancer therapy programs. A whole new resource had opened up for me. In the midst of this remarkable experience, I first came to hear about Dr. Donato Perez Garcia from Mexico City and Donatian Therapy. Following our initial meeting in Montreal, we arranged to get together at his office in Mexico City, where I stayed for a month. During that stay, I witnessed many remarkable instances of patients experiencing relief from their pain and, in many instances, recovery from their diseases.

I knew that many would say, "You're acting crazy!" and "Mexican cancer treatment indeed!" Nonetheless, I also knew of my own experience. Regardless of stereotypes and national prejudices, I knew there was—and still is—something of great value in what I was experiencing. I saw my way clear to doing the work needed to translate this personal experience into a sound scientific reality—a tool to be used to more effectively treat patients seeking help.

Early History of IPT – in Mexico

In 1932, Donato Perez Garcia, Sr., MD (1896-1971), developed Insulin Potentiation Therapy (IPT) for the treatment of human disease. A surgeon lieutenant in the Mexican military establishment, this man's preliminary work with insulin involved an innovative course of self-treatment for an emaciating gastrointestinal problem he had suffered from for years. All previous treatments had failed to resolve it. When he first learned of the then newly discovered hormone insulin for treating diabetes, he noted that in addition to diabetes, this new medicine was also indicated for the treatment of "nondiabetic malnutrition." So, because of his malnourished appearance, he saw it fitting that he should try this insulin treatment on himself. He took injections of insulin before meals, and ate a short period of time thereafter. While the treatment was completely successful with the weight gain, there were times earlier on in this personal medical experiment when his blood sugar would go too low, too fast. His nurses were the only ones present, and they successfully bailed him out with syringes full of hypertonic glucose.

After a few weekly treatments, Dr. Perez's symptoms disappeared and his weight became normal. Reflecting on his experience here, he considered that the insulin had somehow helped his bodily tissues assimilate the food he had eaten. He then went on to reason that insulin might have a similar effect to help tissues assimilate medications. That was his thinking, and it led to a widespread phenomenon of health and healing for many human beings, with remarkable and valuable clinical outcomes.

In his clinical work, Dr. Perez decided to first use IPT in the treatment of tertiary neurosyphilis, the standard treatment for which was relatively ineffective, particularly for advanced cases with brain involvement. Dr. Perez Garcia reasoned that treatment might be improved with the addition of insulin to help the brain assimilate the antisyphilitic medications. Thus, preclinically, an animal study on dogs showed an increased brain uptake of Salvarsan—the arsenic-containing agent used to treat syphilis. This data was published in *Revista Medica Militar* (1938) in Mexico. Subsequently, when applied to his patients with neurosyphilis, Dr. Perez Garcia's treatment was very successful. In many patients, the spinal fluid Wasserman and Lange's colloidal gold reactions were normalized, and there was a concomitant clearing of the symptoms and physical findings in these patients.

In 1937, Dr. Perez Garcia was invited to the United States to demonstrate his therapy at the Austin State Hospital in Austin, Texas, and later at St. Elizabeth's Hospital in Washington, D.C. In 1944, he was again invited to treat some patients at the San Diego Naval Hospital, producing the same positive results in patients with neurosyphilis, malaria, rheumatic fever, and cholecystitis. This 1944 visit to San Diego led to a *TIME* Magazine write-up of Dr. Perez Garcia and what they called his "insulin shock treatment." The commentary from the *TIME* editors read as follows: "Last week Naval Hospital doctors were still scratching their chins about the insulin treatment. But they were impressed by Dr. Perez Garcia. They would like him to come back and do it all over again."

The first successful treatment of cancer with the therapy happened in 1947 when Dr. Perez Garcia reportedly treated a patient with a squamous cell carcinoma of the tongue. This patient subsequently survived—disease free—for another thirty years. Numerous other cancer cases followed, with numerous startling clinical responses—particularly in patients with newly diagnosed disease. There had always been much criticism and controversy surrounding Dr. Perez Garcia and his treatment—fed no doubt by some professional jealousy. Needless to say, the addition of the issue of cancer only served to harden the feelings of many of Mexican physicians against him.

In 1955, Dr. Perez Garcia's son—Donato Perez Garcia y Bellon, graduated from medical school, and joined his father to work at his clinic in central Mexico City. Together father and son continued to expand the applications of IPT to more and more different diseases and, as before, continued to produce remarkable clinical results. And, as with so many medical innovators before them—the likes of Ignacz Semmelweis and Louis Pasteur—Both Semmelweis and Pasteur met with scorn and derision for putting forth what were considered radical, new concepts by the nineteenth century European medical community. Semmelweis postulated that deaths from childbed fever resulted from a lack of cleanliness on the part of the delivering physician, and could be prevented by hand washing; Pasteur challenged conservative tenets of chemistry and medicine. While

Pasteur eventually received acclaim for his efforts, Semmelweis' was largely discredited by his peers and he died - frustrated and angry - of an infection he contracted in an asylum— the excellence and unorthodoxy of the Drs. Perez Garcia earned them nothing but rejection from their peers...

In one instance, this censure came to an extreme. A senior medical student whose professors had told him of the evils of the Drs. Perez Garcia came to confront the two in their clinic. He brandished a pistol with the intention of killing them both for the disgrace he believed they were bringing down on the Mexican medical profession. There were some dramatic moments that night—in a grappling struggle for the gun, it went off—leaving a hole in the ceiling. After subduing him, the Drs. Perez Garcia explained and clarified their position. The young man listened and then left, bemoaning that darker side of human motivation that could create such falsehood and resistance to truth.

In 1971, Dr. Perez Garcia, Sr., died of a stroke. The younger physician then continued on his own—more alone now than before, and more resolved than ever to bring credit and credibility to his father's pioneering work. He himself fared no better with the local medical community, but his many grateful patients continued to thrive, and to refer others, who thrived as well. And so it goes.

Dr. Perez Garcia y Bellon had a son himself—Donato Perez Garcia, Jr.—who earned his MD degree in 1983. In his turn, this youngest of the family namesake undertook the practice of IPT and continued the family heritage of producing remarkable successes with his practice of the therapy in the downtown Mexico City clinic. After several years of partnership with his father, Dr. Perez Garcia, Jr., took himself and his family north to Tijuana where he is currently practicing.

Dr. Donato Perez Garcia y Bellon died of a heart attack in Mexico City on November 23, 2000. His passing was a great loss for the world medical community, as Dr. Perez Garcia was the acknowledged master of the practice of IPT. His dedication to completing the work of IPT started by his late father—Dr. Donato Perez Garcia, Sr.—was total and uncompromising. He accomplished much in this regard. More remains to be done, and will be—by his son, Dr. Donato Perez Garcia, Jr., and Dr. Steven G. Ayre. This is our common dedication. Dr. Perez Garcia y Bellon will be greatly missed.

Developing IPT

In the spring of 1976, having learned what I had about IPT from my month long visit with Dr. Perez in Mexico City, I believed the treatment had value, and I believed that I could play a role in seeing it properly developed for use by the scientific medical community. And so it began. This treatment was about medicine. It involved medicine, and I believed it could be regarded as fully complementary to the existing state of the art in clinical medicine.

I was taught in medical school that liver, skeletal muscle, and adipose tissue were the only tissues that had insulin receptors on their cell membranes. The first time I ever really felt the earth move beneath my feet happened while I was at a scientific presentation on insulin. The presenter made a statement to the effect that insulin receptors were to be found not only on cells of liver, skeletal muscle, and adipose tissue, *but also on cells comprising the ciliary body of the iris*. I felt myself literally shaken by this statement. It challenged the reality of medical understanding taught to and accepted by me.

Misoneism means "the fear of change and the hatred of new things." I now understand that misoneism is the barrier to transformation and growth in the field of medical science—as well as in other functions of our society. Recognizing the challenge that this reality presents is what growth and maturation are all about. I realized that in this matter of the ciliary body of the iris I was participating in a paradigm shift. It was here my medical education took a big sharp turn—up.

I started working on the challenge of IPT in 1976. By 1998, I had four articles published in the peer-reviewed medical literature, made numerous presentations on the scientific theories about IPT at a number of national and international conferences, and had even undertaken two animal studies on the actions of insulin on biomembranes. Though I had shared my understanding of IPT with many practitioners, researchers, and government employees, IPT was still no closer to being available, to any degree, to the general patient population.

Thus, in November 1999, I opened Contemporary Medicine in Burr Ridge, Illinois, a southwest suburb of Chicago. Throughout it all, I had a faith, a belief, that what I was doing was right. I felt it in my heart. I saw it in my practice, and I heard of it in the testimonials and anecdotal patient accounts over the years. Since IPT began use as a cancer therapy in 1946, many thousands of patients have used the IPT therapy to treat their cancers, and to rid themselves of pain and organic dysfunction.

During the eighty odd years of history that tells the story of IPT, all who have had a hand in it have held to the conviction that the therapy is a valuable thing, and that the knowledge of it should be made widely available to the medical profession. Efforts to this end continue. It has become clear that the way to accomplish the desired goals for IPT is to work quietly and diligently, treating those patients who have failed standard therapy, and who have asked for help, documenting all results, and publishing these results in medical journals. See Appendix C for published articles.

As the history of IPT unfolds, so too have the strength and maturity of its proponents. They have come to understand that it does no good to try to push the river, so to speak. The river will flow, ceaselessly, at its own pace. Drs. Perez and Ayre take comfort in the words of the French playwright and poet Victor Hugo, "stronger than all the armies in the world is an idea whose time has come."

It is our dedication to share this dynamic medical process with doctors of medicine in countries worldwide.

CHAPTER 1

How IPTLD™ Saved My Life

By Annie W. Brandt

Presidential Founder and Executive Director of The Best Answer for Cancer Foundation[SM]

Annie was formerly an Executive Software Consultant; a Business Owner; an Indoor Air Quality Consultant; as well as a Founding Member and co-owner of a Green Design/Build Company.

Contact:	**Annie Brandt, Presidential Founder and Executive Director** **The Best Answer for Cancer Foundation**[SM]
Address:	8127 Mesa Dr., B206, #243 Austin, TX 78759
Phone:	512-342-8181
E-mail:	annie@elkabest.org
Web site:	www.elkabest.org

Diagnosis: July 2001 – Advanced-Stage Metastatic Breast Cancer

NOTE TO THE READER: This chapter is for cancer patients, survivors, and interested physicians to help explain (a) why I chose IPTLD™ and (b) why I **_know_** it was instrumental in saving my life. Throughout this chapter, I will insert the **phrase in bold "THINGS I LEARNED DURING MY JOURNEY"** that are followed by ideas and data that the cancer patient may find helpful. Remember, these inserts are based on my

---

research and my observations and are only intended to stimulate thought and open the mind to possibilities.

My story starts nine years before my cancer diagnosis, when I was diagnosed with a dysfunctional immune syndrome. I had to learn how to treat the illness with things other than conventional drugs, as there was no known treatment. I discovered how influential diet, spirituality, mind/body medicine, and vitamins/herbs could be on the body and the immune system. I learned that doctors know only what they learned in school and in "practice," and that there was a whole world of knowledge out there on healing. Between the 1992 diagnosis of the dysfunctional immune syndrome and the cancer diagnosis, I overcame subsequent diagnoses of multiple sclerosis, a heart problem, and multiple chemical sensitivity. By 2001, nine years later, I thought I had my health problems licked!

On the Fourth of July, 2001, I found a lump under my left arm, in my normal wash pattern. The mammogram and the ultrasound did not show anything in my breasts, but my doctor still thought I should have the lump biopsied. I booked an appointment with an oncology surgeon, and she did not think it was anything to worry about either. On Friday the thirteenth of July, I had it biopsied. The oncology surgeon came into the recovery room and baldly announced:

"I'm sorry, it is cancer."

Those words were HUGE in my ears and my mind! I was literally frozen in time. The jolt of fear and disbelief was immense, and all I could think was, "I am going to die." I could not seem to see anything or hear anything or physically feel anything. Looking back, it felt like a true "out of body" experience.

1. THINGS I LEARNED DURING MY JOURNEY: *TAKE CONTROL!*

YOU HAVE TO PEEL THE "CANCER" OFF YOUR FACE AND PULL IT OUT OF YOUR EARS AND STRIP IT OFF YOUR BODY SO THAT YOU CAN SEE AGAIN, THINK AGAIN, MOVE AGAIN. THIS ALLOWS YOU TO TAKE CONTROL OF YOUR LIFE AND YOUR DESTINY, WHICH IS AS IT SHOULD BE.

YOU NEED TO BE THE ONE TO MAKE THE DECISION OF WHAT THERAPY YOU ARE GOING TO DO—NOT THE DOCTOR, NOT YOUR SPOUSE, NOT YOUR FAMILY OR FRIENDS. REMEMBER, IF YOU DIE, THEY WILL ALL STILL BE HERE!

I have spoken to many other cancer patients since 2001, and they all had similar feelings about their reactions to their diagnoses.

- **YOU FEEL AS IF YOU ARE BLINDED.** You feel blinded by the panic and fear; it is as if your eyes are covered over with the word CANCER and you cannot see around it.

- **YOU FEEL AS IF YOU HAVE GONE DEAF.** It is as if your ears are blocked by the words I AM GOING TO DIE, and you cannot hear anything else.

- **YOU BECOME A "DEER IN THE HEADLIGHTS," AS IF YOU ARE WATCHING A SPEEDING CAR COMING STRAIGHT TOWARD YOU, AND YOU CANNOT MOVE.** Your mind and body feel frozen in place. Your heart is beating so fast, and you are shaking inside, and all the stories and "snapshots in time" of people you have known who have been in your situation are running through your mind—most of them bad. You are in a panic to do something NOW, to get rid of this deadly thing that has grown inside you, but you don't know which way to turn.

- **YOU ADOPT THE SHEEP METHOD.** Most peoples' first impulse—mine, too—is to turn to the doctor and say, *"What can I do? What are my options?"* What we are basically saying is, *"Save me. Tell me what to do. I will do whatever you say."* This is what I call the **The Sheep Method**, or **"follow along blindly."** The best illustration about the dangers in this behavior that I have ever come across appeared in the following article from Wiki news (Wikipedia News).

---

450 Sheep Leap To Their Deaths In Turkey

July 8, 2005

450 sheep leapt to their deaths in the Turkish village of Gevas. The chain reaction started when one sheep went over the cliff, enticing nearly fifteen hundred others to follow. According to the Aksam newspaper, by the time the 450 had died, the pile of sheep carcasses at the bottom of the cliff had apparently grown large enough to cushion the fall somewhat, resulting in the saving of the other 1550.

http://en.wikinews.org/wiki/450_sheep_leap_to_their_deaths_in_Turkey.

When I was young, and I wanted to follow the current fashions, my mother used to say, *"If everyone stuck beans up their nose, would you?'"* Well, the answer is *yes* for most people. How many times have we heard **"Go with the flow"?** Or the terms *"status quo"* and *"safety in numbers."* We figure that, if that is what most people are doing, it must be the best thing to do. Not true! Let me give you an example.

GOING WITH THE FLOW IN THE COMPUTER INDUSTRY

As a software consultant in the computer industry, I worked for Digital Equipment Corporation (DEC). We did things slightly differently than IBM, and we were the second-largest computer corporation in the world, right behind IBM. Our systems and software were hands-down better than what IBM produced. The only reason we were second was because *we weren't IBM.* We didn't advertise, so we were not a household name. We hadn't been around as long as IBM, either, so we were the "new kid on the block." We were "different"; we were not the "norm." When people had computer needs, they went first to IBM; the belief was "IBM is the biggest, and most businesses use them, so they must be the best." **Sheep blindly following sheep.**

GOING WITH THE FLOW IN YOUR MEDICAL TREATMENT

You may think: "Yes, but computers are not about life and death. Doctors are not IBM salespeople; they have been through extensive schooling. And I would go to someone very experienced; someone who had been practicing medicine for years."

Actually, even with my nine years of experience with the fallibility of doctors fresh in my mind, those were *my* thoughts. This is the path *I* initially took. I turned to my surgeon, who had just given me the diagnosis, and asked, *"What can I do? What are my options?"* She told me that the recommendation, since the tumor was not readily visible—and that it was at least stage II—would be a double mastectomy instead of a single mastectomy, followed by chemo and radiation. The surgeon told me she could fit me in the following Tuesday for the operation. *And I agreed!* It was that deer-in-the-headlights thing that was happening to me.

So, how did I peel off the "cancer" and take control? I got empowered through knowledge—knowledge is power!

2. <u>THINGS I LEARNED DURING MY JOURNEY: *DO YOUR RESEARCH!*</u>

A person I knew at the time helped me snap out of my nightmare/ sleepwalking state by saying to me, "You are the first person to tell everybody else to do their research and here you are just letting the doctor tell you what to do!" I realized that I had the whole weekend in which to figure out what the doctor was suggesting that I do. Here are some things I found during my research that weekend.

On cancer.

- By the time a tumor shows up, it has usually been growing in the body for up to eight years. *For this reason alone, unless it is a very aggressive cancer, I believe the patient has the time to make an informed decision!*

- Cancer is *smart!* It knows when you are trying to kill it, and it will build immunities to things like chemo. Which is why I am sure you have heard, sometime in your life, the story of someone going through cancer treatment only to have a doctor say, "I am sorry, we have tried all of the chemos, and there is nothing left to offer."

- Regular cells have a birth, a life cycle, and a death; cancer has only a birth, then it lives until its host dies. I often think that this is the only way that cancer is stupid. If it were a really intelligent animal, it would keep the host alive.

- Something everyone should know: cancer LOVES sugar. It also loves stress, negative emotions, fear, and anger—probably because they weaken the immune system, which makes the cancer stronger.

- The immune system cannot see cancer, because it camouflages itself to look like something familiar and harmless.

- If cancer is not growing, it is dying. Its whole purpose is to thrive and grow, so when a cancer remains the same, even if it does not get smaller, that is a powerful sign. It means that you have regained the upper hand in your cancer dance.

On surgery.

- Surgery is an assault upon the body. Anything invasive is just that—you are invading the body. The same holds true here. Surgery causes emotional and physical stress.

- Surgery weakens the body and the immune system. The conclusion you can draw is that anything that weakens the immune system strengthens the cancer.

- It is a medical fact that surgery stimulates cancer, and has been proven to cause metastases.

On conventional chemotherapy and radiation. Both:

- Kill the P53 tumor-suppressor gene, the very gene you need to fight cancer.

- Distort the DNA of your healthy cells, making them precancerous.

- Weaken the immune system.

- Damage vital body organs.

- Cause the cancer to build immunities.

- Have many violent side effects, severely affecting quality of life.

All of the above make the cancer stronger.

After discovering all of this, I decided that I would not follow the conventional path. I felt that, with my dysfunctional immune system and precarious state of health, the conventional methods would kill me. [NOTE: I also confirmed this belief with a second-opinion oncologist.] I decided that, if I was going to die, I was going to go with grace, dignity, and all of my body parts! It was also going to be my decision—I didn't want to ever think I let someone else decide how I was going to live, or die.

On Monday, when I went in for my pre-op appointment, it was to tell the doctor that I had decided against her recommendations. Before I did that, though, I asked her about my research into conventional surgery and chemotherapy. When she confirmed everything I had discovered, I asked, "Why would I want to do that?" She answered, "Because that is the only option we have that offers you a good chance to live." I told her that it was not the only option out there and that I was going to seek other alternatives. She sadly told me that my cancer was advanced-stage, at least stage II but probably more advanced than that, and she did not hold out much hope for me.

I had the double-edged benefit of *knowing without a doubt* that conventional cancer therapy would kill me fairly quickly and unpleasantly. The good news, to me, was that I would not have to try to fight cancer while dealing with all of the side effects of conventional therapy. The bad news was that, whatever I chose to do, I would be doing it against the mainstream of medical experience and knowledge.

At the time I was diagnosed, there were very few people to talk to about their experiences with cancer that had not done conventional medicine. Alternative medicine was regarded with suspicion for the most part. There were not many survivor stories and very few statistics. It was automatically assumed by everyone from my doctors down to the checkout woman at the grocery store that I would be doing conventional therapy. The pressure was amazing, fierce, and passionate.

Additional scans by my oncologist showed lesions in my brain and lungs. They were now saying advanced-stage metastatic breast cancer (I would not let them stage me due to the negative mind/body impact). My oncologist told me to get my affairs in order.

Here is where the peer pressure got almost overwhelming. Everybody I knew was shocked and horrified that I was not going to go straight into conventional therapy. The research that I had done helped tremendously. I was able to point out to them what the dangers were with conventional therapy and the reason why I was not going to do that. There was a general sad-shake-of-the-head and sympathetic expression directed my way each time, while people silently consigned me to the grave. But eventually they left me alone and waited for me to die.

3. THINGS I LEARNED DURING MY JOURNEY: *BUILD A SOLID INTEGRATED HOLISTIC PLATFORM ON WHICH TO PLACE THE CHOSEN CANCER THERAPY!*

So now I knew what I was **not** going to do, but I still needed to determine what I **was** going to do. Back to the Internet and library...

I researched survivors. I found that most of them followed a program. By program, I mean a grouping of elements that make up a whole, coordinated approach.

Over the past several years prior to the cancer, I had already been employing components of holistic therapies for my dysfunctional immune syndrome. These included spirituality, diet and vitamins/herbs, exercise, and mind/body medicine. Now I had to tweak all of those to accommodate a cancer-killing approach, and I added in immune system boosters, lifestyle changes, and a detox program. You can read about the holistic program that I developed and still employ in my upcoming book: *7 Powerful Habits of a Cancer Survivor*.

For the next year, I employed this solely holistic approach with no other cancer therapies. However, in July of 2002—exactly a year after my diagnosis—I found additional swollen lymph nodes. I knew the cancer was on the move again and that I needed to add a formal cancer therapy to my holistic platform.

4. THINGS I LEARNED DURING MY JOURNEY: *STAY STRONG BUT NOT STUPID (or "CHOOSE WISELY, GRASSHOPPER")!*

So, OK, what I had been doing held it off for a year, which was already longer than the doctors had given me! But it was obviously not enough. It is important that you stay positive about your chosen therapy, but do not close your eyes and refuse to see the elephant in the room! If you find that what you are doing is not working exactly as you think it should, examine it *carefully*, get some other opinions, do more research, and consider tweaking the therapy or changing it. I knew here that I had to tweak it. I knew I had to add something very powerful, a therapy that would be hard on the cancer and yet still be easy on my body, my immune system, and me.

WHY I CHOSE IPTLD™

I went back to the Internet and this time I found IPT/IPTLD™. WOW! Here it was! It had all of the components that I was looking for:

- It had a history of being developed in 1929 and *successfully* used on cancer since 1946—it was not "bleeding edge" medicine

- It targeted the cancer, not the patient

- Because it was a targeted therapy, it could use very low doses of the drugs

- It was not harmful to the vital body organs

- It was not harmful to the immune system

- It was not known to cause side effects

How could I have missed it the first time? I could not believe such an elegant, simple, yet sophisticated therapy had been around for over eighty years, used on cancer for 55 years, and yet was not known to the general public and was not a regular offering in oncology!

When I questioned my oncologist, he said that it was considered "experimental" because no clinical trials had been done on it. I questioned that again—why hadn't something this straightforward, simple, seemingly effective, and "friendly" been tested? The only answers I can get to date from the pharmaceutical companies is that the drugs are already FDA approved and to institute the expenses for another trial that actually employs a much lower dose would not be cost effective for them because they would not sell as much chemotherapy!

IPTLD™ is, in reality, an off-label use for FDA-approved insulin and chemotherapy drugs. Many, many medical treatments in this world are, in effect, off-label uses of one drug or another. The theory behind the science of IPTLD™ is that, because diseased cells have more insulin receptors on their surface than healthy cells, a small dose of insulin is enough to stimulate the diseased cells without engaging the healthy cells. At the height of cancer cell stimulation (the therapeutic moment), the chemotherapy is delivered and is taken up by the cancer cell. A dose of glucose completes the treatment. As mentioned before, cancer loves sugar, so the glucose is also taken up by the cancer cells, effectively sealing the chemo in. I think of it as a Trojan horse delivery system for chemo to the cancer cells.

But back to the issue at hand. There were several doctors in the United States who provided IPTLD™, but at the time, there were no IPTLD™ doctors in Texas. I chose to go to Mexico and Dr. Donato Perez Garcia III. I went because, first, my insurance would not pay for an "experimental" therapy, and I needed the affordability that Mexico promised. Second, more importantly, Dr. Donato was the grandson of the inventor of IPT! I was going to the most experienced IPTLD™ physician in the world.

So here was another new experience: I called a doctor and actually got to talk to him personally! [NOTE: this is a characteristic of most IPTLD™ physicians in that they are accessible to the patient in many ways and take a more personal interest in your situation. Almost every IPTLD™ physician will get on the phone with a patient.] Dr. Donato told me that I would need to send him my records and then come for a consultation. He said he would be honest with me as to whether or not he could help me. When I decided I wanted to book my consultation and potential first treatment, he made room for me in his schedule immediately!

His Web site had complete detailed instructions in English on how to get to his clinic and what to expect when I got there. Later on in my therapy, I stayed at the Best Western Americana in San Ysidro, California, because they offered a free shuttle across the border and back, to and from doctors' clinics in Mexico. But the first several times, I took the trolley down to the border, walked across, and hailed a cab. I never had any problems at any time. People were friendly and helpful, the weather and scenery were beautiful.

My consultation and resulting first appointment were on Labor Day, 2002. Dr. Donato said during my consultation that he thought he could help me, although he could not promise me complete healing. He thought he could achieve remission.

Dr. Donato was obviously a very experienced physician, as well as being very knowledgeable about IPT/IPTLD™. But, unlike my regular doctors, he was warm and compassionate and interested. He was not ruled by the clock or in a hurry to get me out of his office. Instead, he patiently sat and answered every question that I had. He asked questions of his own about my lifestyle and eating habits, and we started talking about my holistic program and what he wanted me to tweak and why.

The treatment itself was amazing. I had come in fasting, per his instructions, just in case we decided to do a treatment that day. Another surprise—I did not have to wait days or weeks for another appointment; he cleared some room in his schedule for me! The nurse took my vitals, my weight, checked my blood glucose level and pulse, and hooked me up to an IV. Dr. Donato came in and injected some insulin into the IV, the dose based on my body weight. I began to read my book. During this time, Dr. Donato came in several times to check on me and to inquire how I was feeling. I also received some antibiotics, liver support, antibacterials, and anti-inflammatories via IV and intramuscular injection.

After about twenty-five minutes, I noticed that I was very warm and slightly drowsy. I felt very relaxed, even somewhat "loopy"—I didn't have any interest in reading anymore, but I was still awake, and aware of what was going on around me.

At this point, my blood glucose level and pulse were taken again and it was determined that I was in the "therapeutic moment." Dr. Donato then delivered the chemos into the IV, followed immediately by some glucose, and I was done.

The treatment had taken about an hour. Dr. Donato sent me out for an ultrasound, which was handed to me immediately afterward. I brought it back and Dr. Donato discussed it with me right then. Another huge difference from what I was used to with conventional medicine! My experience with alternative medicine is that it is much more personal and hands-on. He counseled me on what he wanted me to eat that day and from then on. He gave me a prescription for anticancer supplements and an anti-inflammatory drug, booked my next appointment, and I left.

I went out for a light meal and then back to San Diego to do some shopping and sightseeing, to treat myself to some fun. Yes, I had fun during that treatment and every other treatment after that. I felt that the treatments themselves were such a light and friendly way to treat cancer that I needed to continue that feeling in daily life. My research had shown me that laughter and fun would boost the immune system and light up the frontal lobe of the brain, effectively cancelling out fear and proving to be anticancer. Attitude is everything!

I lived a very normal life generally. So I found ways to laugh, because I knew that boosted my immune system. Because I had no side effects from the IPTLD™ therapy, I was able to continue living life as usual, with many "mini vacations" to San Diego/Tijuana for my treatments. I never lost my hair, I never felt sick, I had plenty of energy, and I did no disfiguring surgery. In this way, cancer became a "nonevent" to me, which is—again—another anticancer therapy.

In December 2002, the ultrasound technician finally found the breast tumor. IPT had calmed the breast tissue down enough to see it. It was at 12:00, back against the chest wall, and it was 1.5 cm at that time (Dr. Donato estimated that it had started out in the 3 cm range).

Again, my standard oncologist encouraged me to have a mastectomy, and again I refused. In March 2003, my tests showed no sign of cancer. My oncologist refused to believe it might have been because of IPT; instead, he said "It is probably spontaneous remission!" Today, eight years after I was given my death sentence, my oncologist calls me his little "head-shaker," and continues to be amazed at my health and the quality of life I enjoy.

In July of 2003, I told Dr. Donato that I wanted to do my part to bring IPT/IPTLD™ to the world by establishing a nonprofit foundation to support and promote IPTLD™. I teamed up with another like-minded patient, Rachel Best, in 2004 to create The Elka Best Foundation as a project of a 501(c) (3) called the National Heritage Foundation. It was named in honor of Rachel's mother, who died of cancer in 1980. The Elka Best Foundation name has recently been changed to The Best Answer for Cancer Foundationᔆᴹ.

Unfortunately, in 2006, Rachel passed away of an infection entirely unrelated to her cancer. I then took action to legitimize the foundation as a formal 501(c) (3). As the founder, I set up an organization with a Board of Directors that included me, Rebecca Ayre, and LaMae Weber (my two other volunteer directors), Dr. Steven Ayre, and Dr. Les Breitman (two of the key IPT doctors). We formed a Medical/Scientific Advisory Board and a General Advisory Board. The grandson of the inventor and my doctor, Dr. Donato Perez Garcia III, is our senior medical advisor and a key figure in the organization.

Currently, we are an organization of volunteers with a constituency mainly comprised of IPTLD™ physicians and some of the general public. We have passion and spirit, but we always need more funds and volunteers!

We believe a grassroots movement of patients, survivors, and concerned individuals should start a campaign to raise public awareness of this therapy. Perhaps with enough public interest, the pharmaceutical and insurance companies would agree to endorse this therapy as a standard of care. I believe it is our *right* to have IPTLD™ as a *choice* in the oncologist's office!

For more information, to join as a volunteer, or to make a tax-deductible donation, please go to <u>www.ElkaBest.org</u>. For information on IPTLD™ or to contact one of our board-certified IPTLD™ physicians, please go to <u>www.IPTforcancer.com</u> or <u>www.IPTLD.com</u>.

Portions of the previous are excerpts from my books that are due to be published this year: 7 Powerful Habits of a Cancer Survivor© and Train Your Doctor—or Die Trying! ©

DISCLAIMER
****

The ideas and opinions expressed herein are mine alone, unless otherwise noted.

I am not a medical professional and should not be mistaken for one. I neither diagnose nor treat illness.

CHAPTER 2

Science and Nature in Balance

By Thomas Lodi, MD

Thomas Lodi, MD, has been practicing medicine for twenty-two years. His recent twelve years of specialized training and extensive global experience with cancer patients led him to focus his practice on Integrative Oncology (caring for people with cancer).

For the first ten years of his medical career, Thomas worked in conventional settings as an internal medicine specialist, urgent care physician, and as an intensivist in ICU and CCU departments of various hospitals. Dr Lodi continued his search for more effective and less toxic therapies by training around the world from Japan to Europe to Mexico and all around the United States.

Conditions Treated with IPT: Dr. Lodi uses IPT to treat cancer.
Practice Focus: Teaching the patient how to stop the cancer, treat the cancer itself, and enhance the immune system through nutrition and detoxification.

Contact:	**Thomas Lodi, MD**
	An Oasis of Healing
Address:	210 N. Center Street, Ste 102
	Mesa, AZ 85201
Phone:	480-834-5414
Fax:	480-834-5418
Web site:	www.anoasisofhealing.com
E-mail:	info@anoasisofhealing.com

The WHO (World Health Organization) recently announced that by 2010, cancer will be the leading cause of death worldwide. Only in the past few years have the mortality rates associated with cancer surpassed that of heart disease in the United States and now, after only a few short years, cancer is about to surpass all other causes of mortality on planet Earth. It is unclear whether war has been factored into these statistics but, be that as it may, cancer qualifies as a pandemic of unprecedented proportions.

> What is happening?   Has something changed?
> What is cancer?   Is cancer transmissible (can I catch it)?

Although the answers to these questions are necessary in order to develop a long and enduring therapeutic stance with respect to cancer, the questions themselves beg the involvement of political and economic interests and therefore are not appropriate to our present discussion.

At the very least, it is abundantly clear that nature has become humanity's adversary to be exploited ruthlessly not only without respect, but with a jeering contempt. Consequently, the environment in which we, humans (and all other creatures), now find ourselves, is no longer compatible with health and longevity but rather their opposites, horrific disease states and premature aging and death.

In the United States, one out of two men and one out of two and a half women will develop cancer in their lifetimes. If cancer were genetic, most of our grandparents would have developed, and perhaps died of cancer. Obviously, that is not what occurred and so we must change our investigative perspectives. For example, we now know that epigenetic phenomena are as consequential, if not more so, than the basic genetic makeup of an individual. There is also a huge and rapidly growing amount of data accumulating that indicates that genes are "turned on" and "turned off" by environmental agents, not the least of which are ingested materials, i.e., food, artificial food, poisons, and microscopic organisms.

A bewildering amount of information exists that we do not know or understand regarding this vast subject. What we do know is enough to allow many people with cancer to return to their lives—albeit changed forever. They metamorphose into a condition or state of being more congruent with their human potential than would have occurred had they not journeyed down this road labeled "cancer."

From this perspective, cancer can be viewed as an opportunity and even a blessing since, as we grow toward our potential of optimal functioning, we become an inspiration to those around us. All parents, celebrities, and other role models know a simple fact that we do not teach by what we say, but rather by who we are.

Cancer is simply a word, not a sentence. Autopsies performed on ninety-year-old men find that 100 percent have prostate cancer, although it had not resulted in any disability for the majority of the deceased. Most of these men died from other causes unrelated to prostate cancer. Almost all people in industrialized nations have cancerous cells growing in their bodies but they are of no significant, clinical relevance. Postmortem examinations (autopsies) performed in both Europe and the United States reveal that up to 79 percent of those examined had primary tumors that were either undiagnosed or misdiagnosed while the patients were alive. In one study, 250 malignant tumors were found in 225 patients, and in 57 percent of them, cancer was found to have been the cause of death, although this was unknown while the patient was still living. Simple math reveals that 43 percent of these people who ranged in age from thirty to eighty years of age had cancer although it did not result in disability or death.

The question therefore is not are we going to get cancer but rather, are we going to survive cancer.

It is with this background, along with a deep reverence for nature and an acknowledgement that science, freed from the quagmire of arrogance, atheism, and its illusory fractional perspective, can be integrated with healing modalities derived from both ancient and modern wisdom into a comprehensive program designed to serve as a vehicle for liberation from disease.

Design for Healing Cancer

There are three foundational pillars upon which the healing of cancer depends and which serve to structure the program that we offer at **An Oasis of Healing**:

- Stop making cancer.

- Selectively target and eliminate cancerous cells without eliminating the person.

- Strengthen, rebalance, and empower the immune system.

Stop Making Cancer

Approximately every six weeks, we have new skin; every three days, we have new cells lining our colons; every two days we have new rods and cones in our retinas; every four to six months, we have new livers; and hence every ten to twelve months, we have a new body. Therefore, if we had cancer one year ago and we have cancer today, it is because we are continuing to produce it.

If you put a large scratch in a Rolls Royce, it will eventually rust and corrode. If you are sliced on the arm by a sharp knife, it bleeds, then a scab forms and finally, it heals! Wow! Clearly, this biomechanical earth suit (body) in which we experience our lives, is by far, better designed and engineered than the expensive Rolls Royce. And yet, do we "change the oil, tune it up, or rotate the tires?" NO! But we do expect high performance and are bewildered when we become ill. We even exclaim, "Why me?"

The nature of nature is to regenerate, rejuvenate, and procreate. Just as water runs downhill, so do our bodies heal. If you pick an apple from an apple tree, there will be two or more in its place the following year. If you pull some weeds from the ground, you will find that a tougher brood soon replaces them. Only when nature is prevented from following its course, will healing fail to occur, just as a large dam will obstruct the flow of a river. Remove the dam and the waters will flow. Remove the impediments to healing, and disease disappears. This is the nature of nature.

The two co-conductors of the physiological symphony of life in mammals are the neurological (brain) and endocrine (hormones) systems. And, yes, we are mammals; primates, in fact. Although these two systems are referred to separately, they, as all systems of the body, function as a synchronous, integrated whole.

When two young women move into the same home as new roommates, quite often they find that their menstrual cycles begin to occur at the same time. Obviously, this was not planned. Sharing a living space with someone is very intimate, and just as in other close relationships between people; behaviors, verbal expressions, attitudes, and appetites begin to merge as the bonding between them deepens. This neuroendocrine response is a physiological manifestation of the psychological bonding that the two women are experiencing and indubitably demonstrates the power and reality of thought translating into physiology and biochemistry at a level beneath conscious awareness. Thoughts, from this perspective, therefore, act much like hormones; that is, having their effect on targets at a distance from where they emanate. Since thinking is an involuntary process, it is imperative that we guard, with the utmost vigilance that which is allowed into our minds, just as we would guard that which we are putting into our mouths.

Several glands in the body produce and secrete chemicals called hormones. Hormones have their effect on organs, glands, and tissues, which are located at a distance from the gland. For example, estrogens have their effects on multiple organs, glands, and tissues including the uterus and the breasts. In order for a hormone to have its effect, the target tissue must have receptors specific to that hormone. Then, as the hormone binds to that receptor, specific responses are initiated such as the thickening of the uterine lining when estrogen levels rise during the first part of the menstrual cycle.

The role of hormones is to "turn-on" or "turn-off," that is, to stimulate or inhibit the function of various glands, tissues, and organs. When they are all actively functioning, the body works with a precise harmony and vibrancy seen most abundantly during youth.

All functions of the body other than those hormonally mediated, require nerves to stimulate or inhibit them. That stimulation or inhibition by nerves is a result of chemicals acting on target tissues. Ultimately then, all that ever occurs in the body is chemical reactions.

These chemicals, which mediate life at its most basic level, are produced out of the raw materials that we supply the body when we ingest food or drink liquids. Something worth remembering!

Clearly, it can be seen that an essential aspect to healing requires that the body be restored to a state of hormonal competency through the appropriate use of bio-identical hormones, as well as lifestyle changes.

It is important to realize that hormones do not become "bad," such as testosterone when a man has prostate cancer, but rather the hormones have become unbalanced and the effects of these imbalances produce pathology (disease).

Finally, when one is in a state of health, feeling happy and joyful are aspects of that balance. Therefore, many conditions such as depression, anxiety, and anger, which were thought to be the result of psychological imbalances, are rather the consequences of a toxic, out-of-balance physiology.

Selectively Target and Eliminate Cancer without Eliminating the Person

Cancer Biology

In order to accomplish this requirement, the biology of cancer must be understood. A cancer cell is basically, a defective cell that functions in a primitive manner similar to certain micro-organisms such as fungi (or yeast). What occurs is that a well-differentiated cell such as a breast cell, or a colon cell, or any other type of cell found in the body becomes repeatedly damaged by a variety of causes such as viruses, radiation, chemicals etc... The final insult to the cell, which ultimately distinguishes it from its normal counterparts (normal breast, colon, or other), is that it loses the ability to use oxygen to produce energy. That is, it can only metabolize glucose (universal fuel) for energy through a process known as glycolysis, which occurs in the absence of oxygen. The energy yield from this process is only two ATPs (units of energy) whereas the energy yield from the Krebs's cycle, which utilizes oxygen and occurs in normal, healthy cells, is thirty-eight ATPs. That is a nineteen times (19 X) difference! So, cancer cells are nineteen times less efficient at energy production than normal cells and therefore, in order to survive, they need nineteen times more glucose. That is why we use PET scans to stage cancer. PET scans allow us to locate which cells in the body are taking up glucose (sugar) at a rapid enough rate to be distinguished as cancer cells. The question arises, "How do cancer cells manage to extract nineteen times more glucose from the same blood as a normal cell?" It's quite simple, actually. Cancer cells upregulate (grow) extra insulin receptors onto their surfaces so that they can "grab" insulin quicker, open the glucose channels sooner, and extract more glucose before all the other cells. Well, since that is the mechanism cancer cells depend on for survival, it certainly would be a very strategic mechanism to exploit and, in fact, that is what we do with IPTLD™.

IPTLD™

The person comes into our center not having eaten for at least six hours (usually morning) and is promptly made comfortable in one of our large reclining chairs. After several preparatory intravenous solutions are administered to protect the healthy cells and make the cancer cells more vulnerable, the person is administered a specific, calculated dose of a short-acting insulin. In approximately twenty to forty minutes, all the cancer cells have become saturated with insulin and are therefore permeable (easy passage) while all of the noncancerous cells in the body are only partially saturated with insulin and, therefore, not completely permeable. This is referred to as the "therapeutic moment," which is the time when low dose (approximately 10 percent of standard) chemotherapeutic drugs are administered intravenously. Since the cancer cells are permeable and ready to "eat," they absorb a large portion of the administered dose while the other, noncancerous cells absorb but very little. Because the toxicity associated with this modality is less than 5 percent of standard, the procedure can be performed once or twice a week instead of every two to three weeks as is standard. This allows for tumor shrinkage to occur relatively quickly and therefore any symptoms associated with the tumors, such as pain, partial bowel obstruction, shortness of breath, or limitations of mobility, resolve in a relatively short time. Once the chemotherapeutic agents have been administered, glucose is administered intravenously and the person is given some delicious food to eat. They find that even if their appetite had been dwindling in the recent past, the insulin restores their appetite and they eat quite eagerly and with vigor.

Ascorbic Acid (Vitamin C)

Another modality that targets the cancer cells involves the use of high doses of ascorbic acid (vitamin C) administered intravenously. By achieving specific plasma levels of ascorbates, certain intermediate products of metabolism result that can easily be converted by healthy cells into nourishing substances while cancer cells, being defective and primitive, cannot make those conversions. As a consequence, these intermediate byproducts act as poisons and kill the cancer cells. So, here is a substance that is nourishing for healthy cells and poisonous for cancer cells!

Other Targeting Therapies

There are other modalities employed at our center that also target cancer cells without harming healthy cells. For example, there is a way to block glycolysis (primitive energy production) that affects only cancer cells and other anaerobic organisms such as yeast and anaerobic bacteria. But it has no effect on healthy cells, which utilize oxygen and function at a more sophisticated level.

Immune Enhancement

The immune system has two broad functions; it is the department of defense and the department of maintenance. For this reason, it is imperative to take over as many maintenance functions as possible in order to allow the resources of the immune systems to focus on defense. As will be recalled, most people have cancer even if it has not manifested and therefore remains "silent" (undiagnosed).

It is abundantly clear then, that the avoidance of toxins in our food, water, and air is of paramount importance; hence, not only is it necessary to drive defensively, but also, to live defensively.

We must be ever vigilant as we open our mouths to be sure that we are feeding hunger, not appetite.

Of all the purported immune-enhancing substances that can be found on the Internet and in conversation with others, only a few have been researched and found to be REAL. In addition to utilizing all of the modalities discussed below, we, at An Oasis of Healing, continue to be involved with research from around the world in order to incorporate any and all new advances that are proven to be safe and effective in enhancing immune function.

A rather large body of data has been accumulating from research conducted in Japan as well as the United States and other countries elucidating the immune-enhancing effects of certain **mushrooms**, like maitake, shitake, and agaricus. In addition, certain enzymes in these mushrooms can be used to modify particular carbohydrates found in **rice bran** so that they become immune modulating substances capable of increasing both the number and activity of NK (natural killer) cells, which are responsible for seeking out and killing cancer cells.

In Europe, **ozone** has been used in clinical practice for many years and has accumulated a large body of research to substantiate its efficacy as well as its safety. One of the consequences of using medical ozone on blood is a rather large increase in cytokine and interleukin production by the white blood cells. These are substances that the immune system utilizes to augment immune capabilities and thereby enhance the bodies' defense against cancer, micro-organisms, and poisons.

In Japan, there has been quite a bit of research into a vitamin D3 binding protein that can **activate macrophages** so that they have indiscriminate tumoricidal capabilities. That is, these cells of the immune system (macrophages), when activated, become capable of seeking out and destroying a variety of cancer cells, not just one or a few types.

Finally, there are foods that fuel the immune system and there are foods that fuel cancer. We just have to learn the difference and then modify our appetites accordingly.

Summary

The human body is in constant renewal. It is never static. Billions of new cells are being produced every minute. Billions of old cells, metabolic waste products and poisons from food, drink, air, skin, and lungs need also to be eliminated every minute. When these processes are thwarted, symptoms (body attempting to correct) arise and ultimately, if not remedied, all processes cease.

This is the essence of, **"stop making cancer"** and it is our mission and obligation to teach each of our patients how to stop making cancer. The word "doctor" is derived from Latin and means "to teach." This pillar of the program is, therefore, the foundation upon which all other activities depend at our center. It does not really matter how effective anyone is at eliminating cancer if the person continues to produce it. It is not always difficult to rid the body of cancer; the difficulty lies in keeping it gone!

Cancer cells are defective and have unique characteristics that, when understood, can serve as opportunities to develop strategies that target these cancer cells and preserve the integrity of healthy cells required for optimal functioning (health).

There is a Cure For Cancer; It is Called a Healthy Immune System

Life on planet Earth depends upon the flow of energy from sunlight through plants to animals to micro-organisms. In this transfer of energy from organism to organism, many potentially damaging substances are encountered that would, otherwise damage or destroy those creatures involved, whether they be an oak tree or a human being. Each creature, therefore, is endowed with a system of defense, without which, life would end before it began. This, the immune system, when adequately functioning, keeps all creatures living and when it ultimately fails, life comes to an end. It is abundantly clear then that our activities must be directed toward nourishing and enhancing this system in order to preserve its role as the gatekeeper preventing our descent into death.

Health is the consequence of living in harmony with the laws of nature while disease is the result when those laws are violated. It is very simple. All we have to do is eat fresh fruits, plants, nuts and seeds, sleep early, rest midday, engage in vigorous physical activity, play in the sun, love, laugh, and dance and, above all, be kind.

Healing Journeys

A.T. is a forty-year-old woman who was diagnosed with invasive ductal carcinoma of her left breast in February of 2004. She refused conventional treatment with the exception of oral XELODA, which she began in September of 2008. A.T. had been in relatively stable condition until June of 2008 when she found herself to be continually out of breath with protracted coughing day and night. Upon evaluation by her physician, she was found to have bilateral pleural effusions surrounding her lungs, which compromised her ability to breathe; hence, she underwent several drainage procedures (thoracentesis) and began the oral XELODA.

A PET/CT scan revealed a large left breast mass with extensive involvement of the lungs, pleura, lymph nodes within the chest, bones, and liver. She arrived at our center in October requiring twenty-four-hour oxygen and assistance using the bathroom, dressing, and walking.

At one point, she was hospitalized at a nearby facility in order to receive a blood transfusion and was told by the physicians attending to her that she had no more than two weeks of life remaining.

Eight weeks after arriving in October, she would jog to our center every morning while her husband followed close behind in his car. She no longer required oxygen, was full of energy and joy, was able to attend to all of her own needs, had learned to prepare healthy food and left to go on vacation in Asia.

D.S. was diagnosed with stage IV lung cancer but had refused conventional therapies. He was given a dismal prognosis but being a man in his midforties with a lot to live for, he ignored their soothsaying and found his way to our center. In five weeks, his PET/CT indicated that there was but a small amount of cancer remaining and he opted to complete his program from home in California.

L.G., a sixty-eight-year-old man with chronic lymphocytic leukemia, was diagnosed in spring of 2004. He arrived at our center with a white blood count of 124,000 (normal = 4,000 to 11,000). He arrived in April and by August his white blood cell count was down to 20,000 and he opted to continue his journey back home.

A.M. is a thirty-four-year-old mother of a young girl who came to our center in June of 2008, after being told that she would not live to see her daughter grow and, consequently, she was extremely fearful and desperate. She had been diagnosed with a very aggressive form of non-Hodgkin's lymphoma, which could be seen as a large mass in her abdomen from across the desk during our initial meeting. Her most recent restaging PET/CT in February of 2009 was read as "negative." That is, there was no malignant tissue remaining.

These are but a few of the journeys that we have had the honor to share.

CHAPTER 3

Contemporary Medicine: Healthcare Keeping Pace with Changing Times

By Steven G. Ayre, MD

Dr. Ayre trained with Dr. Perez Garcia y Bellon in 1976 and again with Dr. Perez Garcia in 1997. He is a certified instructor and the Medical Director of Contemporary Medicine.

Conditions treated with IPT: Dr. Ayre uses IPT to treat cancer.

Practice Focus: Offers comprehensive cancer care (IPT, Nutritional Biochemistry, and Mind/Body Medicine) with a kinder and gentler approach.

Contact:	Ayre, MD, Steven G. and Ather A. Malik, DO
	Contemporary Medicine
Address:	322 Burr Ridge Pkwy
	Burr Ridge, IL 60527
Phone:	630-321-9010
Fax:	630-321-9018
Web site:	www.contemporarymedicine.net
E-mail:	info@contemporarymedicine.net

For the times they are a-changin'....
– Bob Dylan, 1963

Contemporary Medicine opened in November of 1999, bringing to reality a carefully cultivated vision that continues to take shape and grow to this day, always striving to combine the best of science with the best of humanity. Medical director Steven G. Ayre, MD, and head nurse Martha Christy, RN, synthesized a growing demand and public interest in "alternative medicine," with a staunchly conservative sense of a physician's responsibility to his or her patient. This sense of responsibility is characterized foremost by a belief that it is the physician's role to translate the gleanings of scientific research and observation, into that which is most therapeutically beneficial to the individual patient. Arising from this belief, Dr. Ayre and now his associate, Ather A. Malik, DO, follow a therapeutic model called Comprehensive Cancer Care, utilizing IPT as the cornerstone of that approach.

Developed by James Gordon, MD, the founder and director of the Center for Mind-Body Medicine, the Comprehensive Cancer Care model is composed of three parts:

1. Something to treat the cancer
2. Nutrition and Lifestyle
3. Mind-Body Medicine or Psychoneuroimmunology

Something to Treat the Cancer: IPT

Dr. Ayre became acquainted with the therapy early on in his career as a physician in 1975 and the results immediately intrigued him. Synchronistically, key studies on insulin receptors in human tissues and cancer cells were to be published over the next several years that verified, in a controlled, scientific context, the empirical findings of the Drs. Perez Garcia. In the following excerpt from "IPT: A New Concept in the Management of Chronic Degenerative Disease," published in 1986 in *Medical Hypotheses*, Dr. Ayre discusses these studies:

> Bar and Roth in their article, "Insulin Receptor Status in Disease States of Man," appearing in the April, 1977, *Archives of Internal Medicine*, state "There are insulin receptors on the classical target cells of liver, adipose tissue, skeletal muscle as well as on numerous other cell types such as placenta, fibroblasts, blood cells and brain."

> As to the question of the functional nature of the insulin receptors on these other tissues, the authors go on in

their discussion to ascribe a characteristically primitive role to this receptor in the cellular physiology of mammalian tissues. In summarizing this, they state that, "The properties of all insulin receptors are remarkably similar, <u>irrespective of cell type</u>."

There is a great deal of empirical evidence accumulated with the Drs. Perez' applications of IPT to indicate that something like such an insulin-permeabilizing and drug potentiating effect does indeed operate in many of the body's tissues. Beyond this simply empirical evidence, it has been scientifically established that the cells making up chronic inflammatory tissue [white blood cells and fibroblasts (2) have insulin receptors on their cell membranes; and as well, certain cell lines of breast, (3,4) melanoma (4) and colon (4,5,6) cancers have similarly been found to possess insulin receptors.

Between 1977 and 1985, medical science confirmed and explored the role that insulin and insulin receptors play in the function of human tissues and cancer, reinforcing what had been demonstrated by the Drs. Perez Garcia over their many decades of practice. Of further interest and relevance were the results of the study "Metabolic modification by insulin enhances methotrexate cytotoxicity in MCF-7 human breast cancer cells," published in the *European Journal of Cancer and Clinical Oncology* in 1981 by Alabaster, O. et al.:

Insulin, which activates and modifies metabolic pathways in MCF-7 breast cancer cells, is shown to increase the cytotoxic effect of methotrexate up to ten thousand fold *in vitro*...This observation supports the hypothesis that tumor cell sensitivity to chemotherapy could be increased by using agents that activate the biochemical or metabolic pathways that determine the cytotoxic process.

While excited and intrigued by the published findings that supported the scientific validation of IPT, Dr. Ayre always emphasized and encouraged the need for further in-depth studies of the therapy.

To this end, he developed relationships with researchers at private institutions and the National Institutes of Health, made multiple presentations in Washington D.C.; Paris, France; and Xuzhou China, and published four more papers on the use of insulin as a biologic response modifier. Still, after a decade of these activities and enterprises, no clinical trials on IPT were conducted. Disheartened, but not discouraged, Dr. Ayre returned to Mexico in 1997 and received further hands-on training in providing IPT to patients from Donato Perez Garcia, Jr., MD, and grandson of the developer, who, since his graduation from medical school in 1983, had been carrying on his family's tradition of providing the therapy.

It took an act of Congress before Dr. Ayre made the transition from being a proponent of the therapy to a practitioner. The Office of Alternative Medicine (now the National Center for Complementary and Alternative Medicine, or NCCAM) was created within the National Institutes of Health in 1991. In August 1997, The Office of Alternative Medicine held a conference in Washington D.C., where director Wayne Jonas, MD, launched a new initiative he had developed termed POMES, which stood for Practice Outcomes Monitoring and Evaluation System. Under this system, nontraditional cancer treatments could be studied in the field on human beings and the information collected could be considered valid scientific data. If a treatment appeared to have promise, a prospective study would be designed and conducted through the National Institutes of Health to evaluate its effectiveness in treating cancer. Dr. Ayre presented on IPT at this conference and returned to the Chicago area equipped with a means and justification for providing IPT to cancer patients in the United States, within a responsible and controlled context.

Over the ten years that he has been providing IPT to cancer patients, Dr. Ayre has never wavered in his conviction that the therapy is of inestimable value in the management of cancer. With its low side effect profile, IPT has proven to be an ideal means of delivering chemotherapeutic drugs to people with cancer, making the therapy an ideal facilitator of Comprehensive Cancer Care. IPT patients look and feel good while in active treatment, leaving them available to focus on the other aspects of self-care involved with Nutritional Biochemistry and Lifestyle and Mind-Body Medicine.

Nutrition and Lifestyle

The program of nutritional support for enhancing immune function recommended for patients at Contemporary Medicine includes advice on food choices and recommendations for nutritional supplements. Our nutritionist, Jim Golick, LDN, CCN, will counsel you on what to eat, what to avoid, and which dietary supplements will support your body in enhancing your immune function and detoxifying your systems of that which does not support healthy function.
Jim describes his philosophy and approach thusly:

I believe in the principle of biochemical individuality, which requires different approaches with each person. As a result, I might utilize blood type and body type principles as well as lab work to arrive at an understanding of your needs. Cancer and cancer treatments present other unique challenges, which I also take into consideration.

I specialize in reducing cravings for junk food, improving mood, energy, sleep, and digestive disorders. I offer ideas for those with high levels of stress, as well as tips on how to eat more healthily in today's fast-paced society. My goal is to work with you to discover simple, yet achievable options to maximize your success.

The First Consultation

The first visit begins with an overview of a symptom and diet survey form (which the staff provides to take home and fill out). We then go over the report and evaluate how well your body is functioning, which foods to eat and avoid, and recommendations for supplements tailored to your needs. A basic detoxification program may also be encouraged. These recommendations will help balance your system for maximum energy and immune strength.

While there is some debate and inconclusive data on the significance and importance of nutrition and lifestyle in relation to cancer, there is no doubt that it *can* be significant and that eating well and exercising regularly will lead to an improved quality of life. Food choices involve nothing that is new or strange—it's mostly good common sense. The quality of one's food intake is as important for health as is the attitude of the heart while consuming it. For it is said, **"The man who eats beer and franks with cheer and thanks will probably** be healthier than the one who eats sprouts and bread with doubts and dread."

Mind-Body Medicine: Psychoneuroimmunology (PNI)

What is Mind-Body Medicine?

Mind-Body Medicine is the practice of medicine based upon the scientific understanding of the biochemical underpinnings of awareness and consciousness. In their book *Cancer Report*, authors John R. Voell and Cynthia Chatfield clarify it as the practice of medicine with an understanding that the "mind and the body are one, and that our emotions and feelings are the bridge that links the two."

Put simply, in the words of Candace Pert, PhD, body and mind are "flip sides of the same thing." When managing and treating illness and disease, the condition of both the mind and the body must be addressed as they are one and the same.

Candace Pert, PhD, the neuroscientist whose groundbreaking work created the foundation for Mind-Body Medicine as a science, remarks on the relationship between the mind and the body:

> We might refer to the whole system as a psychosomatic information network, linking psyche, which comprises all that is of an ostensibly nonmaterial nature, such as mind, emotion, and soul, to "soma," which is the material world of molecules, cells, and organs. Mind and body, psyche and soma. (Chatfield, Voell 65)

The Science of Mind-Body Medicine

The scientific basis for Mind-Body medicine was established through the work of Candace Pert, PhD. Over the course of fifteen years, while heading a laboratory at the National Institutes of Health, Pert published over two hundred scientific articles developing the concept of neuropeptides and their receptors.

Pert compiled the results of her work in the book *Molecules of Emotion: The Science Behind Mind-Body Medicine*. First published in 1997, this book explains human feelings and emotions in terms of chemical happenings that can be measured within time and space.

These happenings are physical interactions between molecules called neuropeptides and receptors. Most significantly, Pert explores how the interaction of these powerful molecules affects our immune system and our body's relationship to disease.

Uniting Mind and Body

Pert's research is revolutionary in terms of Western scientific trends. The Western mind has long relegated emotions and feelings to a place separate and outside the realm of science and medicine. According to Pert, seventeenth-century philosopher Rene Descartes instituted this schism of mind and body.

In the article, "NIH Challenged to Integrate Alternative Medicine," which appears in the online edition of *Psychiatric News*, author Richard Karel describes a hearing on Capitol Hill, titled "Healing and the Mind." Pert, one of the panelists, explained that in order, "to get permission to use cadavers for dissection, <u>Descartes had to promise the Pope</u> that he wouldn't have anything to do with the soul, the mind, or the emotions—those aspects of human experience heavily under the church's jurisdiction—but would stick strictly to the physical." The result of this agreement, she expounded:

> **Set the tone and influence for the future of Western science over the next two centuries, dividing the human experience into two distinct and separate spheres that could never overlap, creating the lopsided mainstream medicine we know today.**

By gathering measurable, quantitative data proving the existence of human emotion, Pert united what was once put asunder by the "Cartesian Split." An example of the "Cartesian Split" would be: body-mind, matter-spirit.

The Application of Mind-Body Medicine: Lawrence LeShan, PhD, and Susan Silberstein, PhD

Lawrence LeShan, PhD, is a clinical and research psychologist with over fifty years of experience in counseling cancer patients. Over those fifty years, he has achieved extraordinary results.

According to *Cancer Report*, "Approximately half of his cancer patients with poor prognoses have experienced long-term remission and many are still alive decades later. Nearly all these patients dramatically improved their emotional state and quality of life (133). He is the author of several key books, indispensable in the genre of Mind-Body Medicine and cancer. Most notable of these are *Cancer as a Turning Point: A Handbook for Cancer patients, Their Families and Health Professionals*; *You Can Fight for Your Life: Emotional Factors in the Treatment of Cancer*; and *How to Meditate: A Guide to Self-Discovery*. Additionally, he has been honored for his work in the field of psychotherapy with the Gardner Murphy Award (American Society for Psychical Research), the Pathfinder Award (Association of Humanistic Psychology), and the Norman Cousins Award.

A Joyous Approach

In his approach to psychotherapy, Dr. LeShan seeks to bring out what would give his patients the most joy and fulfillment in their lives. In his words, the emphasis of the work is on "What is right within me? What brings me joy and a sense of purpose in me?" He seeks to guide his patients on a path of inspiration and discovery. He seeks to generate in them a sense of excitement and enthusiasm for the life they live.

The psychotherapy approach taken by Dr. LeShan is by no means meant to cure cancer. Rather, it serves to augment whatever course of medical treatment, conventional or alternative, that a patient has chosen. The therapy is meant to mobilize an individual's immune system and give him or her a reason to make life worth getting out of bed for in the morning.

To summarize his approach, "Getting cancer can become the beginning of living. The search for one's own being, the discovery of the life one needs to live, can be one of the strongest weapons against disease." Counseling sessions and workshops with Dr. LeShan and his associates are available through www.cancerasaturningpoint.org.

The Center for Advancement in Cancer Education (CACE)

In 1977, Dr. Susan Silberstein founded The Center for Advancement in Cancer Education (CACE) upon the death of her husband at the age of thirty-one from cancer. In the fulfillment of her mission to help others who experience the pain and uncertainty of cancer, Dr. Silberstein has counseled more than twenty-five thousand cancer patients, relying solely on tax-deductible donations.

In addition to her counseling services, Dr. Silberstein has dedicated her energies to a multitude of projects. Notably, she has presented at many national and international conferences on mind-body and nutritional topics in the approach to cancer care. For more on Dr. Silberstein and her efforts, visit the CACE Web site.

Mind-Body Counsel

In counseling sessions with her clients, Dr. Silberstein is sensitive to certain emotional or environmental patterns that could be contributing to an individual's malignancy. She develops counseling sessions around the idea that thoughts and emotions directly affect an individual's immune system.

She stresses, however, that while it might be evident that a client in some way contributed to the development of his or her disease, she deals with this subject in an innovative way to avoid creating feelings of guilt and stress. In an interview with Silberstein, as published in *Cancer Report*, she describes her approach:

> If you tell patients they have a "responsibility" for creating their illness and their wellness, it implies some blame and leads to guilt. If you spell it the second way, "Response Ability," you create an awareness that leads to power. This second way can lead to opportunities for the awareness of many theories, research results, and clinical observations relating to emotions and behaviors that might control or reverse their illness. (111)

We all have an ability to respond to the circumstances that rise up in our lives. How we respond is entirely our choice. Mind-Body Medicine is about helping one harness the inherent power and freedom in personal choice.

Dr. Silberstein also acknowledges that not everyone will survive cancer and that is an issue that is acceptable within the expanded parameters of Mind-Body Medicine. In her interview from *Cancer Report*, Silverstein shares:

> Some patients just want to let go and be with a loved one who has passed, we help them to die spiritually at peace because they have gotten in touch with where their spirit

really is. Because sometimes it has already crossed over long before the body goes and that's ok. (111)

When applied to our perception of human disease, the tenets of Mind-Body Medicine allow for an infinitely expanded understanding of who we are as living beings. Disease is an opportunity for growth and self-discovery, not something to be feared. Death is a passing from this form of existence, not a failure. Mind-Body Medicine allows us to embrace life on its own terms.

Mind-Body Medicine Counseling at Contemporary Medicine

Our life coach, Teresa McGrath, provides gentle, caring, and inviting hands to hold your heart. She listens carefully and provides understanding wherever you are at. She guides you to move forward on your path to improved emotional and spiritual health. Since mind, body, and spirit are all intertwined, you will find your best results by addressing all of these aspects, not just the physical. Her intention is to significantly improve the quality of your life, which often helps your physical health as well.

Some of the processes that Teresa utilizes are:

- Spiritual Growth: Creating peace, love, and joy in your life. Understanding the purpose of life. Gratitude and prayer work.

- Identifying the message that your illness is trying to bring you.

- Deep relaxation/meditation/visualization. These tools promote emotional and physical peace, which stimulates your immune system to function optimally for the benefit of your health.

- Forgiveness Work: Many people say to "Forgive and Forget." But, how do you forgive? Using the lessons of Byron Katie, acupressure, spirituality, and Radical Forgiveness, she will guide you to "let go" of that unhealthy baggage that can slow down your healing.

- Affirmations and the identification/removal of obstacles.

- EFT—Emotional Freedom Technique. This is a simple acupressure technique that anyone can learn. It dramatically and quickly dissolves negative emotions that can be very harmful to your health.

- Emotion Code: This is a muscle testing technique to identify and release personal and inherited trapped emotions.

Contemporary Medicine

Just what is contemporary medicine? It is based in the concept that the physician serves as a guide for the patient as he or she charts a path through life, holding forth an image of health and well-being when the patient is not able to conjure a sense of these things for him or herself. In part, it is a departure from a naïve fervor and fascination with science, that it will somehow save humanity. It is an understanding that science will not save humanity, but that science and humanity are one and the same. It is an understanding that **humans are more than the sum of their parts, and the human experience cannot be reduced or confined to a collection of biochemical happenings, cells, and organs subject to infallible manipulation by pharmaceuticals, nutraceuticals, or any other sort of remedy.** It is a departure from the confines of reductionist thought and a move toward looking at health and life creatively, and from multiple perspectives.

In a message to his patients titled, "Managing Malignancy: Our Answer to Cancer," Dr. Ayre concludes:

> The ultimate responsibility to be faced in one's personal war on cancer, as well as the ultimate paradox in it, is to be able to accept "come what may" out of the efforts you make—either with gratitude, or with graciousness. Either kind of clinical outcome here—be it a "success" or be it a "failure"—comes with its own mark of victory. Put another way, 'it is possible for people to be healed without being cured.'
>
> In victory, these experiences thus being equal, I would opt for success and for joy and for love in this life. This medicine of effort, when done and worked at, becomes

the medicine of joy. All the staff at Contemporary Medicine and myself offer you our prayers and our very best wishes for these things in your life.

Perhaps the end of death from cancer will come not from any one innovative or revolutionary drug or treatment, but from the combined efforts of the patient and his or her physician, working together with respect, dedication and love for one another, their families, and their planet, to create a new world through an inspired sense of purpose.

இஇ

CHAPTER 4

My Story

By Richard Linchitz, MD

Distinguished medical doctor, author, lecturer, and outspoken expert on health issues: Dr. Linchitz balances the demands of running a private medical practice in New York with requests for his straightforward analysis of complex medical matters in television, radio, and print media.

Known as an inspiring speaker, educator, and man of extreme compassion and vision, Dr. Linchitz's presentation style offers a message that's both practical and wise. His unconventional techniques have been adapted from his own personal health victory and more than three decades of research, culminating in a book that is currently in development. For inquiries on booking Dr. Linchitz, send an e-mail to daureen@gmail.com or call 301-996-6020

Contact: Richard Linchitz, MD, Linchitz Medical Wellness PLLC

Address: 70 Glen Street, Ste 240
Glen Cove, NY 11542
Phone: 516-759-4200
Fax: 516-759-7600
Web site: http://linchitzwellness.com
E-mail: rlinchitz@msn.com
Training Date: Trained in 2005 with Dr. Perez Garcia.

Conditions treated with IPT: Dr. Linchitz uses IPT to treat cancer.
Practice Focus: Performs Chemo-sensitivity testing along with nutritional counseling, detoxification, and energy medicine for a personal patient program.

This chapter is dedicated to our patients, whose quiet courage serves as a source of constant inspiration.

In order for the reader to understand the rationale for our comprehensive anti-cancer regimen, I would first like to share my own personal experience with cancer.

In December 1998, after a routine exam for an unrelated condition, my doctors found a cancerous tumor the size of a large lemon in my right lung. I had never smoked and was always athletic so I was understandably shocked by the diagnosis. Gradually, the shock turned into a mission to understand the nature of cancer and help others find their own path to healing. In the early days and weeks after my diagnosis, I realized that my previous responses to my patients who found themselves in similar situations were incomplete. In the past, I would have immediately advised patients to contact an oncologist and put themselves in his or her hands. When it came to my own condition however, I began to doubt that advice. When I looked into the available treatments, I realized that for a minimal proven benefit, I would face treatment that would seriously compromise the quality of my life. There did not seem to be any traditional medical resource that could help me discover the underlying reasons for my cancer. There were also no traditional resources to help improve my strength and resistance to the disease that was threatening to take my life.

I gradually came to realize that truly comprehensive cancer treatment should include a two-pronged approach. One prong would be to find an effective way of killing cancer cells without destroying the immune system and without destroying the overall health and integrity of the body. The second prong would be to actually improve the health and cancer-fighting ability of the body through what I came to call "The Six Pillars of Vibrant Health."

I will first describe the six pillars and how they are integrated into a comprehensive approach to cancer care, and then go into more detail about effective techniques of killing cancer cells.

The first pillar of vibrant health is our diet. In cancer this takes on an even more urgent importance. Cancer cells, like most cells, require glucose to derive energy. However, cancer cells, because of their more primitive and inefficient anaerobic metabolism, require much more sugar than normal cells just to survive. If they are to maintain their rapid growth pattern they need that much more sugar. All our cells take in sugar through a mechanism that can be conceptualized as a "lock and key" system where insulin is the key and an insulin receptor is the lock. It turns out that cancer cells have many more "doors" with these "locks and keys" than normal cells. This is understandable because any cancer cell without a mechanism for concentrating sugar will not survive. Only those cells with high concentrations of these receptors will be able to rapidly divide and develop into cancerous tumors.

Conventional physicians are aware (or should be) of this mechanism and even use it to help diagnose cancer with the PET scan (positron emission tomography). Its theory is very simple: a radioactively labeled sugar is injected into a person's vein. The sugar travels through the body and causes the body to produce insulin. The insulin "keys" then attach to the receptor "locks" on all the body's cells and the "doors" of the cells open. Cancer cells, however, will have many more "open doors" and therefore will concentrate the sugar with the radioactive tracer. The body is then scanned for radioactivity and the cancer "lights up" on the scan.

If we think about this process carefully, does it tell us anything about the way we should eat? Of course we should limit (or preferably eliminate) our sugar intake and our intake of anything else that will cause a significant rise in our blood sugar (especially refined carbohydrates but even sweet fruits and grains can be a problem in some patients). This is essentially the same diet we recommend for our diabetic patients. In fact, there is an association between diabetes and prediabetes with high blood sugar and insulin levels on the one hand and with cancer incidence on the other hand. We also know that rising blood sugar interferes with immune function.

We also need to eat organic food to limit the toxins entering our body. We must also be careful to limit our intake of omega 6 fats which are pro-inflammatory and pro-cancerous. We should increase our intake of omega 3 fats which are anti-inflammatory and generally anticancer. The proper balance of these fats fights inflammation and cancer. We must avoid trans fats or partially hydrogenated fats, which are pro-inflammatory and interfere with cellular communication and with the transport of nutrients. In short, a whole food diet, focusing on lots of vegetables (mostly raw) with organic, naturally fed (grass for cows, grass and worms for chickens) animal products (free-range chickens and eggs, wild salmon, grass-fed beef, raw milk, kefir and cheese, etc). Recent studies have shown that the right diet can improve survival rates for several cancer types.

The second pillar is supplements. Many supplements have been shown to have anticancer effects in preclinical studies and some even in clinical studies in humans. Some have been shown to be powerful immune stimulants (such as the various mushroom products). Others have been shown to have direct effects on cancer metabolism causing cancer cells to die. At Linchitz Medical Wellness, we have developed a protocol of natural agents that interfere with cancer angiogenesis (cancer blood vessel formation). If cancer cannot make blood vessels, its growth and ability to spread would be severely limited. This is the theory behind conventional agents such as Avastin but the natural agents work through many mechanisms. This protocol could even potentiate the effects of agents like Avastin as well as classic chemotherapy drugs. There are other natural agents that have been shown to potentiate conventional chemotherapy drugs by increasing their penetration into the cancer cells and by interfering with the ability of the cancer cells to become resistant to these drugs.

Exercise is another crucial pillar. Recent studies have shown improved survival rates in patients battling cancer as well as improved quality of life. Exercise can be thought of as a continuum between activity and rest, both of which are important. Overtraining can be just as destructive to immune health as inactivity. We have found that the most effective exercise program is the one that patients are willing to follow. It can be walking, swimming, yoga, weight lift training, etc. Ideally, short bursts of intense activity with longer periods of rest or easy activity in between, will provide optimal immune stimulation and will be manageable for most patients.

Stress can play an important role in interfering with immune health, in causing inflammation, and in disrupting hormonal balance. The forth pillar, stress management, is a general term under which spirituality and living with meaning or purpose can be included. At Linchitz Medical Wellness, we encourage patients to meditate, to pray, do yoga, tai chi, or anything else that gives them relaxation, peace, and a sense of inner strength. We also use "quantum biofeedback" and "EFT" (Emotional Freedom Technique) to help reduce stress and improve emotional balance and well-being.

The fifth pillar is detoxification, a subject curiously ignored in conventional medicine. Heavy metals, for example, are known immune disruptors and many of them are frankly carcinogenic. Those patients with body burdens of these substances need chelation to help restore immune competence and cellular energy. Pesticides, plasticizers, and many other environmental toxins are endocrine disruptors and have been implicated in the rising incidence of breast and prostate cancer as well as other types of cancer. In addition to chelation, at Linchitz Medical Wellness, we offer far-infrared sauna treatments and colon hydrotherapy to aid in the detoxification process. The first pillar, a clean diet, will also limit toxin exposure. Vegetable juicing and eating high-fiber food will speed elimination and detoxification as well.

The final pillar is hormone balancing. One important example of the hormone problem is the growing epidemic of unrecognized hypothyroidism. It has been recently noted in studies that breast cancer is associated with high TSH values (a symptom of hypothyroidism). Hypothyroidism suppresses immune function in general. Many patients have cancers that are sensitive to hormones. In fact, it is sometimes the presence of higher levels of toxic estrogen metabolites (like 4.- OH and 16-OH estrone) that may have predisposed the patient to cancer in the first place. Fortunately that thyroid gland can sometimes be naturally stimulated (in some cases the removal of toxins from the body can aid this process). For other patients, replacement of thyroid hormone is indicated. In the case of toxic estrogen metabolites, diet change and simple supplements and exercise can lower these levels. There are other hormonal issues that can also play a role. All must be taken into account in order to optimize treatment.

We have covered the six pillars but what about aggressively killing the cancer cells that have appeared in our body? Insulin Potentiation Therapy LowDose™ chemotherapy (IPT) is an effective, yet gentle way of killing cancer cells. The theory behind IPT could not be more logical. Cancer cells in general concentrate sugar through their abundance of insulin receptors as described earlier. If a small measured dose of insulin is given, the cancer cells become selectively more permeable, then the insulin receptor sites are maximally saturated with insulin (the therapeutic moment). Very small doses of chemotherapy agents are then introduced into the body and these doses are effectively concentrated into the cancer cells providing enhanced killing powers with a much lower side effect profile.

How do we choose among different chemotherapy drugs? As with conventional oncology, we can choose an agent that has been shown to be effective in most patients with a specific type of tumor. However, in the interest of a truly individualized approach to treatment, we can send the patient's blood to a laboratory in Europe that will test the blood for circulating tumor cells and then test these for resistance to various chemotherapy drugs. This will allow us to pick out the most effective drugs for each individual patient. These drugs could be very different from the standard protocols in oncology. This laboratory will also test for alternative (natural or nontraditional) agents that can help overcome chemotherapy resistance or even directly kill cancer cells. Natural killer cell function (a measure of immune function) is also assayed (tested) and information is given as to the most effective agents to more effectively attack the cancer.

We often use high dose vitamin C intravenously as part of the overall regimen. This can be combined with vitamin K3 (which has been shown to potentiate (make stronger) the cancer killing effects of vitamin C). The National Institutes of Health is currently studying high dose vitamin C and has shown it will kill most cancer cells when given in high enough concentrations (these concentrations can be achieved only with intravenous vitamin C).

There are many other potential treatments available, some of them very innovative. All treatments are individualized to each patient with the goal of maximizing benefit. As new research emerges, we are constantly updating our protocols to offer the most effective treatments.

CHAPTER 5

The Odyssey of a Cancer Patient

By Constantine A. Kotsanis, MD

Constantine Kotsanis, MD, is one of the early U.S. physicians to embrace Integrative Cancer Therapies. Introduced to IPT therapy in 2001, he trained with Dr. Perez Garcia. Dr. Kotsanis is a certified IPT/IPTLD™ instructor.

Dr. Kotsanis graduated from the University of Athens Medical School and completed residency in Otolaryngology from Loyola University of Chicago in 1983. He is Board Certified in Otolaryngology-Head and Neck Surgery, a fellow of the American Academy of Otolaryngic Allergy, and licensed by the Arizona State Board of Homeopathic Medicine. He is a certified Clinical Nutritionist. Dr. K. has been a practicing physician for twenty-five years. As Medical Director of the Kotsanis Institute, he conducts research, treats and educates physicians and patients alike. His mission is to change the way health is delivered to the world *one person at a time*.

Contact:	**Constantine A. Kotsanis, MD**
	The Kotsanis Institute
Address:	2020 W. Highway 114, Ste 260
	Grapevine, TX 76051
Phone:	817-481-6342
Web site:	www.kotsanisinstitute.com
E-mail:	info@Kotsanisinstitute.com

Training Date: Trained with Dr. Perez Garcia in 2001.

Conditions treated with IPT: Dr. Kotsanis treats cancer, chronic resistant infections, and chronic fatigue with IPT.

Practice Focus: Treating the patient based on the individual's physical, metabolic and biochemical makeup. He combines nutrition counseling and anti-aging therapies for different ailments.

Introduction

Cancer is a disease of the immune system that deserves special attention. The literature cites no less than one hundred reasons for the cause of cancer. However, the most profound cause is related to lifestyle! What the patient is seeking is a compassionate physician, who is willing to navigate through the maze of the physical and emotional concerns of a suffering human being. Physicians and families are some times too quick to pass a death sentence on the afflicted. I find this behavior unacceptable as a physician and as a human being. Patients and doctors need the correct information. With correct information all things are possible including cancer cures. I foresee in the near future that most if not all diseases will have a cure. Understanding the solid scientific principles of nutrition, detoxification, biochemistry, biophysics, and psychology is a prerequisite to conquering cancer.

As a treating IPT physician, I believe we must have depth of knowledge in all disciplines of medicine. Understanding of Western medicine, homeopathy, acupuncture, naturopathy, structural medicine, integrative medicine, functional dentistry, and nutrition is a must for an IPT physician. However, this covers only the bare necessities of a scientific understanding of cancer. Because dealing with cancer is complex and emotionally charged, it is crucial that the IPT physician studies and understands the dynamics of the patient's relationship with his or her family, friends, working environment, and financial ability to complete recommended treatments. Everyone involved must be willing to dedicate the time and energy of fulfilling all tasks.

The Odyssey of a Cancer Patient

As a cancer patient one must consider at least seven parameters before seeking out IPT and other integrative therapies.

Advantages and Shortcomings

First and foremost, **one must understand the advantages and shortcomings of IPT therapies**.

Susanna is a fifty-year-old female with inflammatory breast cancer diagnosed for the first time in January 2008. The patient said that prior to her diagnosis she was a fairly athletic individual with a reasonably healthy lifestyle. She stated that her stress level was minimal, with the exception of the death of her parents eight years ago. She is self-employed, unmarried with no children, and overall a happy individual. There is no genetic information because she was adopted.

Conditions include a lot of dental problems with multiple mercury fillings and problematic root canals. She states that in her twenties she had several severe infections. She also had severe recurring tonsillitis and was placed on many antibiotics for a great length of time prior to a tonsillectomy. Blood tests done elsewhere also show toxicity to aluminum. The patient was first diagnosed with swelling under her left arm in the fall of 2007. Diagnostic tests confirmed a stage III-B breast cancer. Her traditional oncologist recommended chemotherapy followed by radiation. The patient chose to bypass traditional Western medicine altogether and began several alternative treatments on her own. These alternative treatments included Protocel, vitamin B17 and alkaline and organic foods. Despite these self treatments the problem continued to worsen.

In October of 2008 she visited our clinic for the first time seeking IPT. On examination her left breast was inflamed and necrotic with redness and inflammation. She immediately began IPT treatments twice a week and eventually once a week. The IPT treatments were tolerated well with the exception of one episode of nausea; she also had slight hair loss, which she attributed to her hypothyroid hormone status. Once her hypothyroid status was corrected, her hair was restored. By late February of 2009 she had received twenty-five IPT treatments and had tolerated them very well. Before and after IPT, PET scans revealed that, with the exception of a couple of small lesions on the surface of her breast, she was negative for cancer. The breast and the area around the skin was almost completely healed. The consistency of the breast tissue was normal. At that point she felt that the disease was completely resolved and for financial reasons she decided to begin self-treatment again. She felt that she was "cured" from the disease. Our clinic did not agree with her assessment. We advised her to continue IPT at least once a month along with solid nutritional treatments and close observation. Despite our recommendations the patient stopped all follow-up in our clinic. We referred her to an oncologist and primary care physician for a second opinion; however, she did not follow through. By May of 2009 she reported by phone that her cancer had returned and now it was worse than it was before. She was again advised to visit our clinic for a full evaluation but for financial reasons she has chosen to enter a traditional oncology research protocol closer to her hometown.

Susanna's treatment with IPT, although very successful initially, failed to provide a long-term solution because she did not understand that once you are diagnosed with this disease, you must follow medically supervised treatments for life. In my clinical experience patients like Susanna have done well with continuous treatment with IPT and the natural and nutritional treatments when they stay with a lifelong program.

Like Your Doctor

Second, patients must choose physicians they like. Just remember, a good physician will offer you appropriate therapy. A great physician will serve you for life! Eugenia is such a patient. She matched her personality with all the doctors she came across. She was first diagnosed with breast cancer in April of 2006. She first noticed a discharge from her nipple and felt a lump in her left breast. Her oncologist officially diagnosed her with breast cancer and recommended a traditional approach to her disease. However, she chose help from a semi- traditional physician in 2006. He recommended mastectomy followed by his special therapy. The patient refused surgery and allowed only a special oral protocol by this physician. In conjunction with the proposed protocol she was also treated with IV Herceptin, a target drug for HER2+ cancer; however this caused undesirable cardiac side effects. Three months into the treatment of the initial three tumors, one had disappeared completely and the other two had reduced in size. Due to financial and emotional stress she decided to stop the treatment.

For the next year and a half the patient was self-treating with multiple supplements such as DHA, D-aromatase, amino acid drops, and other natural products. In January of 2008 the PET scan showed that her breast cancer was in stage IV. She reported that a large lesion had developed in her left breast beginning in October of 2008. For this she self-treated with topical colloidal silver solutions. Her traditional oncologist recommended topical therapy with Flagyl to keep the infected wound under control. Her oncologist told her that there was nothing else he could do at this time.

In early February of 2009 she visited our clinic for the first time. She reported generalized fatigue, pain to her breast and chest, and inability to sleep and work. The initial physical examination revealed that the entire left breast had a large gapping split all the way down to the chest wall, with induration necrosis, and putrid odor secondary to severe localized infection. What was encouraging about Eugenia was her spirit and her willingness to live. Because of her fighting spirit and the support of her loving family we decided to work with her for potential life extension with minimal morbidity.

Our initial goal was to control the raging infection and to reduce her pain. For this we introduced a special treatment that modulates pH and ORP (oxidation- reduction potential).This amazing but simple technology takes advantage of the basic principles of biochemistry and biophysics. It is designed to change the pH and the ORP of all body tissues. All degenerative diseases have an acid pH and a positive ORP. The normal healthy cell has an ORP of -70 mV. As disease progresses, the ORP slowly drifts toward -30mV. All cancer shows a -30mV ORP and an acid pH. Normal tissue pH approximates that of the blood (pH 7.414). This method very quickly restores the normal ORP and the normal pH of the tissue. In less than thirty days the patient has a feeling of well-being again. In short, this intervention acts as a gentle but very powerful antioxidant without any significant negative side effects.

The pH and ORP manipulations managed to strengthen Eugenia to the point that she could withstand surgical debridement of her necrotic breast. She was referred to a plastic surgeon to perform debulking of the disease by removing the breast and a primary closure. After surgery we had minor setbacks from the original infection. Cultures from the draining wound revealed pseudomonas infection. Under the supervision of an infectious disease physician she received intravenous infusions of antibiotics. Within three weeks the infection was completely resolved and the surgical wound was completely healed.

Once she was stabilized, we started IPT. We also we performed a special blood test from Germany that tested for the drug sensitivities of tumors. Once we received the test results from Germany, we chose the most appropriate chemotherapeutic agents and used the IPT principles to continue IPT treatments. By the end of April 2009 she had receive ten IPT treatments and had tolerated them well. Although the physical exam and her feeling of well-being seemed to skyrocket, a repeat PET scan after the tenth treatment showed stabilization of the disease without regression.

Eugenia, being very optimistic, wanted to press on with additional integrative approaches anywhere in the world. She wanted to beat her disease and see her children grow! Off she went to London, UK. She traveled there to seek a new experimental treatment. This treatment is also designed to target only cancer cells, a similar concept to IPT. With this treatment the patient ingests a patented form of chlorophyll. This chlorophyll is selectively absorbed by all the cancer cells in the body. Then they use a special ultrasound technology that activates the chlorophyll to destroy the tagged cancer cells. This concept is similar to IPT therapy, which also selectively destroys diseased cells. One- or two-week sessions are enough to accomplish potential total destruction of active cancer cells. She went to London and received this treatment in May and June 2009. She returned to our clinic and continued her aggressive nutritional and pH and ORP treatments. So far she has done very well clinically, with minimal complications. Her quality of life has been excellent. She is always in good spirits when we see her.

This extensive workup and treatment of Eugenia shows that one can achieve quality life extension with minimal complications. At the center of this philosophy are the willingness and understanding of the patient and the physician to leave no stone unturned. The credit to the success so far belongs to Eugenia and her loving family. Although we do not know the long-term outcome of her comprehensive treatments, the patient and her family are happy with the results at this point. These results are much kinder and more humane compared to entering a hospice program back in January of 2009, as recommended by her primary care physician. Love, hope, persistence, and exploration of all possibilities is what has kept Eugenia alive, happy, and productive to date.

Third, one must dedicate the time needed to get healthy and stay healthy; this is a lifelong commitment. Margaret is a natural health professional that strongly believes in the mind-body-soul connection. She is truly a pleasant, well informed health practitioner about all aspects of medicine. Although she is not totally against Western medicine approaches, she favors natural healing and natural medicine. She first visited our clinic in October of 2008 with a history of inflammatory breast cancer on the left side. Ten years prior she had a similar breast mass on the right side that she was able to heal using natural botanicals, vitamins, and nutritional manipulations. Despite her diagnosis of breast cancer she decided initially to self-treat until

March of 2009. Due to the increased discomfort and slow progression of her disease she visited our office seeking IPT as well as all other supportive therapies.

We decided to begin an aggressive antioxidant program (pH and ORP manipulations), along with correction of thyroid dysfunctions and correction of emotional stressors. For the emotional component we referred her to an integrative psychologist who was able to address her emotional issues. Within a few visits to this psychologist, the patient felt a significant change for the better. She felt as if "the cancer had left her body."

Based on the biochemistries done at our office along with the sensitivity test from the German lab, we successfully controlled and significantly reversed the disease clinically to the point that she feels normal. Margaret understands that the fight is not over and also understands that she needs to continue persistent aggressive treatments for life. For this, she has agreed to continue IPT once a month for the next year, as well as all nutritional and emotional support as recommended by all her health care practitioners. We anticipate life extension for this patient with excellent results.

Fourth, one must make permanent changes in nutrition for life under the supervision of your IPT physician or a clinical nutritionist. Grace is a fifty-two-year old female who presented to our clinic in January of 2009 with stage IV estrogen receptor-positive metastatic breast cancer. She was first diagnosed in November of 1994 with a lump on her right breast during a self-exam. She was diagnosed with stage I cancer confirmed by biopsy. The history included a lot of stress in her life, the terrible Western diet, along with a sedentary lifestyle. She had several root canals with mercury fillings for many years. She also had a history of chronic infections as a child and many yeast infections as an adult.

In March of 1995 she underwent a mastectomy on the right side and received a total of six intensive chemotherapy treatments by a traditional oncologist between June and August of 1995. She had lost all her hair and had frequent nausea from the treatment. She did not receive any radiation therapy. The patient said she was led to believe that chemotherapy would prevent the recurrence of any cancer in the future. However, a year later she discovered a lump on her left breast. Her oncologist told her she was simply suffering from paranoia and not cancer. She visited a surgeon who preformed a biopsy followed by mastectomy. This was also malignant. Until 2005 the patient had no complications, no symptoms of cancer, and no other treatments. Then in 2005 she began to experience severe pain across her left chest as well as along the left side of her rib cage. The chest X-ray of the area proved to be unremarkable. However, the bone scan showed something suspicious. The patient dealt with her pain for nearly two years and received only cortisone shots from time to time. In March of 2008, a repeat bone scan at M.D. Anderson Cancer Center indicated that she indeed had a recurrence.

By April of 2008, the patient was diagnosed with stage IV, non-curable breast cancer. The patient began making drastic changes to her diet, including eliminating almost all sugar intake. She also began taking supplements of B6, flax oil, and barley tablets, as well as juicing organic vegetables. In June of 2008, the patient's oncologist started her on a medication called Xeloda, an oral chemotherapy drug. The patient stated she took this medicine for only a couple of days, complaining of both mouth sores and hot flashes. Later that month, the patient traveled to Mexico where she received high doses of IV vitamin C, oxidative therapies, and UV light therapy as well as vitamins K and B17. She credits these treatments with building her immune system. After returning to the United States, the patient again started Xeloda, this time with more success. She was also given monthly IV treatments of Zometa.

At the end of 2008 she decided to explore all known treatments, integrative and traditional. By the beginning of 2009 she had opened the Pandora's box to alternative and integrative medicine. Her traditional oncologist had left her with little hope and very few options for her disease. When she first visited our clinic in January of 2009, she was intrigued by the combination of IPT and natural healing. Her extremely supportive husband and family encouraged her to follow her heart's desire to conquer her disease. She began reading books about natural healing. At my recommendation, she read *The China Study* by Campbell. This completely changed her mind about life and nutrition. She is perhaps the most compliant patient when it comes to following instructions. *The China Study* primarily focuses on a raw vegan diet. Although she is not 100 percent a raw vegan, she has eliminated all nonorganic foods, most animal food products, and sugars. She claims that this change has made a significant improvement in her health. In addition to the nutritional changes she also received the pH and ORP treatments in our clinic. The first thirty days of treatment in our clinic included the nutritional changes and daily administration of the pH /ORP program. Within just three weeks, her health and her outlook on life had improved dramatically. At this point, we started IPT treatments. We also performed the special blood test from Germany that showed the drug sensitivities of the ca cells. Once we received the test results from Germany, we chose appropriate chemotherapeutic agents to continue targeted IPT treatments. By mid April 2009 she had receive ten IPT treatments and had tolerated them very well. A repeat PET scan after the tenth IPT treatment showed improvement of her problem. She is now beginning to spread out the IPT treatments every two weeks and will eventually go to once a month.

This is the model patient, medically and emotionally. She really gets it. She completely comprehends the body-mind-spirit connection and has utilized this information to the max. She reports that her friends and the health care providers in her hometown are surprised with her recovery. This proves that good science and a great attitude can defeat or contain any and all disease.

Fifth, one must accept the recommended IPT therapies without being stressed out about making lifestyle changes at this stage of my life. Elizabeth is a sixty-nine-year-old female first diagnosed with breast cancer in April 2007. The patient said that prior to her diagnosis, she was a fairly healthy individual; however, she stated that during Christmas of 1999 she was plagued by an overwhelming amount of stress, which she feels may have been a contributing factor to the development of her cancer. The patient first noticed a painful, swollen lump in her left breast. A biopsy confirmed the presence of multiple malignant tumors, however, the patient states that her cancer has never officially been "staged." The patient refused her physician's adamant recommendation for traditional chemotherapy and radiation; she decided to do her own research and start with self-treatment by changing her nutrition. The co-morbidities (complicating factors) are that she works full-time at a job she describes as "stressful." She has financial strain and worries about a socially troubled child.

She first came to our clinic in January 2008. She was blessed with an "angel" who donated funds for her IPT treatments. For the emotional and stress component of her condition we referred her to an integrative psychologist who was able to address her emotional issues and help her to manage and reduce stress. Once these issues were addressed, IPT treatments were under way. We also performed the special blood test from Germany that showed the drug sensitivities of her cancer cells. Once we received the test results from Germany, we chose the appropriate chemotherapeutic agents using the IPT principles to continue IPT treatments.

The patient did not notice any adverse side effects during any of her IPT session. However, she did advise us that she was able to discontinue her pain medications with the treatment. The patient stated that, in conjunction with IPT, she also introduced barley green tablets, juiced organic vegetables, and nutritional supplements into her diet regimen. She eats mainly organic foods and has limited her sugar intake. After her twentieth IPT treatment, one resilient tumor remained. Upon my urging, the patient agreed to a mastectomy of her left breast. On September 8, 2008, the patient underwent surgery and a total of four lymph nodes were removed, all of which were cancer free. The pathology reports showed that the remaining tumor was completely contained, which the patient attributes to her IPT treatments. To date, the breast has healed completely, with no evidence of any tumors or cancer. The patient states that she is feeling well, gained weight appropriate for her height and she is vibrant, glowing, and very optimistic to live the rest of her life cancer free.

Sixth, one must understand the financial implications involved with any long-term therapies, including IPT, with any threatening illness before getting started. Too often I see patients that stop medically supervised treatments because of financial distress. As soon as they begin to feel better, some patients take it upon themselves to continue home treatments without medical supervision. All too often this approach has undesirable complications. We can refer back to Susanna who chose to discontinue IPT and supervised care despite her great success with IPT. Patients can suddenly find themselves in a much tougher war, trying to fight this alone. At this point, Susanna has experienced a full-blown return of her disease. This may have been avoided if she continued receiving medically supervised care, along with monthly IPT treatments. Following the patient with supervised care is critical in fighting this very dynamic disease. Again it is worth repeating that once you have been diagnosed with cancer, lifelong follow-up is necessary.

Seventh, and last but not least, **one must aggressively explore all treatment options for life!** This brings us to Walter, who is a sixty-six-year-old male diagnosed June of 2006 with stage IV non-small cell adenocarcinoma of the lung with unfavorable prognosis. He is a smoker of many years, retired from a fulfilling career to enjoy gardening at home. He is happily married to a very supportive wife.

The initial PET scan showed two tumors, one in the upper quadrant of the left lung and one in an arterial lymph node directly above the heart. He was initially treated with conventionally recommended chemotherapy and radiation, which was only partially successful with complete reduction of one of the tumors, but with life-threatening complications due to an allergic reaction to one of the chemotherapeutic medications. He decided to explore other options.

Walter is the twenty-first-century Ferdinand Magellan. He is prepared to go to the ends of the Earth to find treatments that work. So on with his world tour. First stop was Germany. There he received a special vaccine made from his own cancer cells. This kept the disease in remission for some time. However, several months later, a repeat PET scan showed a new tumor in the right lung. He then sought IPT treatments at our clinic in November of 2007. He received a total of twenty-six treatments from November of 2007 through June of 2008. Although IPT kept the disease in check, he decided to explore additional new treatments. His second stop out of the United States took him to South Korea. There he received autologous stem cells and cytokines. This finally reversed his disease completely and there is now no evidence of tumors. Thus, the twenty-first-century Magellan was rewarded with complete remission! According to Walter, he is "feeling great and enjoying life and his garden." This proves that persistence, good science, and good luck often can bring very desirable results.

Conclusion

The journey to recovery needs participation from all concerned, i.e., from the patient, family, physician, and staff. Open this new chapter in life with a focus on the things that are important, leaving behind the stress of work. Spend far less time worrying over the little things. Keep an open mind. Approaching any disease with love and compassion will lead to very desirable outcomes for all involved.

"We have seen the enemy and it's us." Researchers have confirmed over and over that most advanced diseases are lifestyle related. Most if not all diseases are preventable. More than anything else, food seems to have a major impact on which diseases we get. Not surprisingly, cancer is underwritten by inflammation and oxidation. Both of these processes are controlled by the foods we eat. **"Let food be your medicine. Let medicine be your food."** **—Hippocrates.**

CHAPTER 6

Why I Chose IPT Treatments

By Charles Gray

My particular cancer was diagnosed in June of 2006. PET/CT scans revealed that I had two tumors, one in the upper quadrant of my left lung, and one in an arterial lymph node directly above my heart. Both tumors were relatively small in size, but subsequent biopsy indicated that the cancer was non-small cell adenocarcinoma, common for heavy smokers, and deadly. My resident oncologist wrote a letter to my family physician, stating that I most likely had less than one year and a half to live, based on normal progression of the disease, but of course recommended that I undergo chemotherapy and radiation to delay the course of the disease.

Being both naïve, and having total trust in conventional medical doctors, I agreed to undergo radiation and chemotherapy. The radiation treatment was somewhat successful, in that the tumor in my left lung was completely eradicated; however, the tumor above my heart was still in force and effect, although it appeared to be destroyed, according to the first PET scan after initial treatment. The chemotherapy treatment was complementary to the radiation, but very nearly resulted in my death, because I was highly allergic to Taxol, and experienced the classic allergic reaction, which is much like a full-blown heart attack.

At any rate, I went into the classic "remission" stage for my type of cancer. Subsequent investigation on the Internet, and information from various friends and relatives, all seemed to lead to one unfortunate conclusion—MY REMISSION WOULD BE ONLY TEMPORARY, as my particular lung cancer was almost always fatal—no known cure. To an old country boy like me, this was beginning to be unacceptable.

I was fast getting tired of people treating me like I was on my death-bed and hearing "I'm so sorry" over and over again. Also, and for the life of me, I do not know why people do this, but I had to listen to the gory and horrific stories of some family member, or friend, dying of cancer. All this only spurred me to investigate every resource known to mankind. I was suddenly on a mission...find a way to whip this disease. I just was not ready at this time to have breakfast in heaven (or possibly worse).

I firmly believe that the good Lord watches over his ignorant children, for it was not much later that a friend of mine at the church I am a member of, told me about an acquaintance, a famous Hollywood movie director, that had an incurable cancer but had received treatment in Germany. He was utilizing a doctor that would be considered "alternative" in the United States. My friend gave me his phone number, and on a whim and a prayer, I called him. It was not long before he called me back. Our conversation was the shortest in my remembrance. He gave me the name of the clinic in Germany and told me that if I had a single brain cell, I would not waste any time getting over there for treatment. I thanked him, contacted the doctor in Germany, and was soon on my way over. I did not know what to expect, but was surprised to receive the level of treatment that I did, including a vaccine made from my own cancer cells that was supposed to inhibit the progression of cancer. After a few months, and still being in remission from the cancer, I made another trip back to Germany to receive more vaccine, but the treatment did not seem to be as effective as before, and shortly thereafter, a PET scan revealed that the tumor above my heart was back, along with a new tumor in my right lung. A quick visit with my local oncologist resulted in perhaps the most discouraging moment in my entire life. I was dying, and there was absolutely nothing he could recommend to help me. No more chemo!

OK! That was it. I determined then and there to forgo conventional medical treatment if all they could do was to tell you to enjoy the rest of your life, as short as it might be. Another friend that I had met in Germany told me of an alternative doctor practicing in Rowlett, Texas, which was fairly close to my home location, and that this doctor had access to a lab in Greece that could tell someone, based on a blood sample, what drugs might be effective against his or her cancer. Off I went! This doctor was straightforward and recommended various supplements to aid in the overall battle against the cancer. He promised no cure, but in the treatment process, received a report back from Greece that stated my cancer was still sensitive to vinorelbine and cisplatin, two chemotherapy drugs. In passing conversation, he said, "Wish I still was able to do IPT, since that might really make a difference in your treatment." Well, it did not take long for the rat to smell the cheese, and I immediately asked, "What in the dickens is IPT?" The subsequent description of the IPT process suddenly hit home. This was a process where the lethal chemotherapy drugs could actually kill cancer cells without serious dose-related side effects, mainly because they are not administered in such large doses, and the good Lord knows that I was already suffering from chemo side effects from conventional therapy, mostly nerve damage to my feet and legs.

Home to research IPT. I found out that the IPT process was discovered by a doctor in Mexico, who used it quite successfully to treat a number of diseases, including cancer. I contacted his son in Mexico, and discussed treatment options with him, but eventually decided to seek treatment from Dr. Kotsanis located in Grapevine, Texas. Thus began the third phase of my cancer treatment—IPT.

After IPT: As of September 2009 (more than three years since his diagnosis), Mr. Gray continues to be cancer free, active, and healthy. After he finished his regimen of IPT he went to South Korea for stem cell therapy, which reconstituted his immune system.

CHAPTER 7

Who Dies? Who Survives? Who Thrives?

By Hendrieka "Hennie" Fitzpatrick, MD

Dr. Hendrieka "Hennie" Fitzpatrick received her medical degree from the George Washington University School of Medicine in Washington, D.C., in 1981. She completed her residency at Case Western Reserve University and was board certified in Family Practice Medicine in 1992.
Prior to becoming medical director of Integrated Health Medical Center, she provided medical care for the underserved as the physician in charge of the "Healthy Tomorrows" Mobile Van, sponsored by Presbyterian Medical Services in Santa Fe. A pioneer medical doctor in the United States for European Biological Medicine, she teaches physicians nationally.

Contact: **Hennie, Fitzpatrick, MD**
              Integrated Health Medical Center
Address: 1532 Cerillos Road, Suite A
              Santa Fe, NM 87505-3512
Phone: 505-982-3936 Toll Free: (866) 690-4975
E-mail: henniefitzpatrick@gmail.com
Training Date: Trained with Dr. George in 2004.
Conditions treated with IPT: Dr. Fitzpatrick treats cancer and other diseases with IPT.
Practice Focus: Strengthening and rebuilding the body through a combination of treatments based on bio-dentistry, nutritional analysis, and deep detox.

Meet Molly: Transcendent Or Crazy?

I entered the exam room on a beautiful day, knowing only that this was a new patient who called to schedule with some urgency. I saw a pale young woman who was no longer just slender, but gaunt.

She was forty-five and the single mother of two children who were sixteen and twelve. She explained quietly that her breast hurt. This shy young woman was hesitant to show me the "sore spot," explaining that the problem had intensified suddenly. She was worried that I would be angry or offended.

In fact, Molly's breast had been replaced by a gaping black hole, oozing a greenish fluid with no identifiable nipple or uninvolved skin. For weeks she had been stuffing the hole with Kleenex and the old tissues had hardened into a rocklike lump.

Despite my compassion for Molly both as a woman and a physician, her wound and the odor of rotting breast was almost unbearable.

In medical school, I was taught to assess the problem, make a diagnosis and a treatment plan for the patient, and to do it quickly and with certainty. I was also taught to distance myself from my own visceral reactions, to judge the situation and make a pronouncement about what is to be done. I was also trained to "tell the truth" to the patient, which encouraged me to calmly state that there is "nothing left to do" or that the only hope is through drastic and death-defying treatment.

With that as my initial medical training, I had gone on to develop a different approach with patients. So I stepped forward, touched Molly's shoulder (instead of recoiling from her dreadful wound), and looked her in the eye. I sat down close to her; I welcomed her to my office and invited her to tell me all about her journey with cancer.

Seven years ago she had been diagnosed with breast cancer after finding a small lump in her breast. As she looked for medical care, she was horrified by the approach of each oncologist she consulted.

She felt vulnerable and abused by their quick and uncaring predictions of her future and she felt "run over" by the impersonal way in which they informed her about chemotherapy, surgery and radiation. And at the beginning, she had felt very well physically.

She wanted to do a lumpectomy and then work to get well with supportive treatments. But the oncologists insisted that surgery could not be done without chemotherapy first. To Molly these oncologists were relentless and unwavering with their opinions. <u>"Abusive"</u> was the word she used.

Overwhelmed, she had consulted a specialist in energy medicine who had convinced her to dangle crystals over the breast lump for twenty minutes twice a day, to stop thinking any negative thoughts, and to never ever allow anyone to say the word cancer in her presence.

Molly worried that her cancer was growing, spreading and invading her chest wall. The healer reassured her that these were good signs of the cancer naturally exiting her body. When she consulted me (which she did because she wanted my help to get rid of the odor and to gain weight), she requested that I never say "cancer."

Physician, First Do No Harm

It is easy to think that this woman was just plain crazy and eccentric. As a physician, I have vowed to always help people who come for help. Regardless of whether she was crazy and eccentric or misguided and frightened, my job is to offer my expertise and help people to get well in whatever way they can accept.

Molly and I worked together for over a year. With an individualized plan, her breast began to heal and she regained her strength. She kept reminding me how she could not believe that I really cared about her and she would not waiver from her belief that the cancer was actually "exiting "through her skin. She chose to refuse all X-rays or other scans.

Eventually she developed severe shortness of breath, refusing to have any hospital evaluation. She finally had no choice and presented to the ER gasping for air. She died of metastatic disease the next day. So deep was her denial that her children were left alone that night, coming home from school to an empty house. The children had no idea their mom was really sick, much less on the brink of death, and were orphaned.

A careful history revealed no family history of breast cancer, no previous significant medical illness; she had been a vegetarian on an organic diet. She had a deep spiritual connection that she relied on to transcend the signs from her physical body, which was disintegrating from cancer.

Evaluate Past Traumatic Events

There is no real difference between the psychosomatic and physical body. Cancer obviously affects the physical body and the most sophisticated medical care requires evaluating the patient's ability to manage cancer and to recover.

To do this requires evaluating past life events for two reasons: first because events dating back to early childhood definitely determine the integrity of the immune and the endocrine systems and secondly because if you, the physician insist that you have the time to listen to your new patient's history, you maximize his or her chances for a positive outcome.

Stress and reactions to traumatic stressors change the physical architecture of the brain. This physical structuring then determines the amounts and rhythms of biochemicals, which determine overall health. To heal from any serious illness requires support of the entire body. Just targeting the cancer is ineffective. So intake history must include detailed information.

Ask about birth and early childhood trauma. Early neonatal experience indelibly sets the stage for every aspect of a person's internal and external functioning. Girls who were sexually or physically abused have a statistically significant increased risk of developing breast cancer because adrenal hormone patterning (hypothalamic, pituitary, and adrenal gland) directly determines immune and female hormone health. The earliest interaction of the mother with her infant sets a lifetime pattern of the balance in the autonomic nervous system.

Ask about dental and medical trauma. These questions elicit the "physical" history (e.g., dental fillings, orthodontia, and tonsillectomy) as well as somatic experiences caused by medical or dental care.

If a new cancer patient has had a bad experience with the initial diagnosis and treatment of cancer this will affect compliance and the outcome of therapy through the neuroimmunoendocrine system(s).

Ask what it was like to be a teenager. The process of puberty—both physical and emotional processes—is another critical time in developing the strength and integrity of the adult psychophysical systems.

Ask about what gives the patient joy and how often does she or he laugh, sing, or relax and play. This is not just a "friendly" question.

The ability to manage the stress of healing from cancer depends on a strong and balanced autonomic nervous system. Joy, laughter, leisure, and a strong network of people you can absolutely rely on, ensures that a person will not just survive, but thrive.

Why Does Trauma Matter?

There are many permanent structural changes in the brain from life stress. We hold in our bodies the residues of everything that has ever happened to us.

Traumatic experiences impair verbal memory. This means that telling the story of the degree of stress from a stressful event is often not possible.

At the time of any stressful situation, the sensory system responds to a programmed trigger with a reaction stored "automatically" in the unconscious memory. The reaction to the stress is automatic and is imprinted by the accumulation of early experience.

The familiar example of this is Pavlov's dogs that were given meat just after a bell rang. The dogs both heard the bell and salivated at seeing the meat. After repeating this sequence of the bell ringing and the presentation of meat several times, the dogs salivate when the bell rings even if there is no meat.

As expected, though, if the bell rings several time and there is no meat, the dogs stop salivating at the sound of the bell. Salivation was imprinted quickly an extinguished quickly.

But what if instead of meat the bell rang as the experimental subject receives a painful electric shock? The imprinting is the same: after several trials the bell will be associated with a painful experience. But if the stimulus (the bell) is associated with a shock, the body reaction will never be extinguished. This means that the cascade of stress responses, which tax every organ system, will always occur in response to the bell even if the electric shock is eliminated.

Traumatic stress reduces the size of the hippocampus, which is a part of the limbic system. The hippocampus receives information from the amygdala and encodes new information as memory. Biochemically, information storage and reaction to the information occurs through the balance of the ANS (autonomic nervous system) and levels of neurohormones and neurotransmitters. Hormone and neurotransmitter levels are ultimately responsible for the ability to recover from any illness. Traumatic stress creates a sense of disintegration that is not easy to verbalize. This sense of disintegration causes irreparable damage to the entire body over time.

Traumatic experiences cause symptoms such as brain fog, lack of focus or motivation, fatigue and depression. These "emotional" kinds of experiences are commonly associated with trauma. Trauma is also a DIRECT cause of: peptic ulcers, coronary artery disease, hypertension, hypothyroidism, immune dysfunction susceptibility to infection, and type 2 diabetes.

Finally, a thorough history of past trauma is important for treatment planning because getting diagnosed with cancer causes an enormous stress to every physiologic system. Seeking alternative treatments and mindfully planning your own treatment path adds another stress, particularly if well-meaning family members are not supportive. Our society perpetuates a rigid belief system around cancer. We all "know" that cancer will shorten one's life and that the treatment for cancer causes suffering. Allopathic medicine coined the term "war" against cancer; indeed, the treatments turn the patient's body into a battleground, pitting the body against itself in a bloody fight for survival. Furthermore, many people feel shamed, guilty and disempowered by the cancer itself. If the patient had many past experiences that caused shame, guilt, or disempowerment, a skilled physician must know this as he or she plans a treatment.

Testing for the Physiological Effects of Traumatic Experience

The initial intake for each IPT patient has to include a careful history of traumatic events. I have developed a questionnaire that I will provide to anyone interested. I encourage you to add or change questions so that this part of cancer care continues to develop. Depending on the office staffing, a staff member may be the best person to discuss these questions and take a detailed history.

Evaluate adrenal, thyroid, and gonad hormone levels, neurotransmitter levels, and always evaluate precise levels of bowel flora. Many integrative physicians agree that hormones are best evaluated by salivary or urine testing as opposed to blood levels. Test kits are readily available, user friendly, and easy to interpret.

Evaluation of the adrenal cortical level requires four to five specimens collected during a single day because the amounts as well as the rhythm of cortisol production are vitally important. Without adrenal repair and rebalancing, IPT outcome will not be optimal. Cortisol levels as well as the daily cortisol patterns directly influence immune system strength, insulin resistance, and thus glucose tolerance and Ig A levels, which are the first line of defense of the immune system.

Proper thyroid evaluation requires measuring T3, T4, TSH as well as a thyroglobulin panel. Healthy thyroid levels are essential for maintaining energy and well being. The normal level of T3 is ten times higher in the brain than in the blood of happy individuals. Any stress that triggers the "fight or flight" response increases cortisol demands; persistently elevated cortical releasing factor (CRF) decreases conversion of T4 to T3. So stress decreases access to metabolic energy and depletes T3 levels. T3 has a role in the suppression of oncogenes (genes related to creating cancer) as well as in viral transcription and creating cellular energy.

Sympathetic nervous system overload occurs from stress, which stimulates inflammatory kinases. Over five hundred different kinases have been identified that affect gene expression. Increased local or systemic cortisol stimulates immune suppression of the B lymphocytes and causes an imbalance in TH1 / TH2 immune systems. Balance of these two arms of immunity is crucial for getting rid of cancer. Finally, stress stimulates angiogenesis, which increases the ability for cancer to grow new blood vessels and therefore spread.

Without adequate levels of thyroid and adrenal hormones, reproductive hormones can also never be properly balanced.

Comprehensive stool analysis provides necessary information for a comprehensive IPT protocol. Bowel flora imbalance results from both a systemic stress response and dysbiosis (pathological colonies of intestinal bacteria) of the gut. With intestinal dysbiosis the ability to absorb anything taken by mouth is compromised. That means that a physician can prescribe a pristine oral regimen of food and supplementation which cannot be properly utilized without healthy bacterial flora.

Probiotic supplementation without a stool analysis is of little use since there is no way to predict the pattern of dysbiosis (imbalanced bacteria) without analysis. Many patients with severe dysbiosis have no intestinal symptoms and report good digestion and bowel habits. Gut bacteria is important to adequate production of serotonin, since most of the serotonin produced is made in the gut. Adequate serotonin levels are needed to maintain a good mood, which is very important, but serotonin also plays an important role in maintaining a healthy immune system.

The physical interdependence of the neurological, endocrine, and immune systems necessitates that any cancer care treatment include an evaluation of all of the systems; this dynamic balance is always profoundly influenced by what has come before in the patient's life experience.

Conclusion

Any physician, but particularly those of us who offer a scope of alternative therapies realize that there are mysterious factors that define who recovers and continues living and who dwindles and dies. These factors are not really so mysterious and need to be evaluated.

The difference in outcome does not depend only on the type or stage of cancer, the treatment protocol, or even the person's compliance. There are other factors that directly affect the ability of a patient to recover. In order to truly design and implement any cancer protocol, a skilled physician must understand these factors and their impact on the course and severity of an illness.

Factors such as diet, exercise, and nutrient balance, and gut health, immune and endocrine health are very important and are commonly included in the original work-up and treatment plan. But in order to predict and then determine cancer treatment outcome, an evaluation of past life events is crucial.

We hold in our bodies a residue of everything that ever happened to us. The endocrine and neurological circuitry that is in place at the time of the diagnosis of cancer directly impacts the strength of the immune system the ability to absorb food and maintain weight as well as the ability of the ANS (automatic nervous system) to endure the treatment without developing side effects.

I find that if I explain these predictive factors to my patients as physiological truths and then address the physiological residues of past traumas I can guarantee a much more positive outcome from IPT treatment.

Being diagnosed with cancer is enormously stressful. We have a deeply ingrained cultural belief that a cancer diagnosis greatly increases the risk of dying of cancer and not old age. The belief system also teaches that the treatment for cancer inevitably involves drugs, surgery, and radiation that causes terrible illness in the name of a cure. Another way to say this is that we all know that you have to suffer in order to possibly get well and that there are no guarantees. It would be one thing if the oncologist told you that you need chemo and radiation and that these treatments mean that you will be weak, bald, nauseated, and vomiting for a year but that then you will be well. It is entirely another thing to understand that you will be weak, bald, nauseated, and vomiting for a year and these therapies may or may not be successful.

CHAPTER 8

Insulin Potentiation Therapy: Mike's Case

Frank Shallenberger, MD, HMD

Dr. Shallenberger has been practicing medicine for twenty-five years. He graduated from the University of Maryland School of Medicine and received post graduate training at Mt. Zion Hospital in San Francisco. He has practiced IPT since 2002. He is one of only sixteen physicians in Nevada licensed in conventional medicine as well as alternative and homeopathic medicine. This allows him to integrate the best of both approaches for optimal results.

Contact: **Frank Shallenberger, MD, HMD**
The Nevada Center
Address: 1231 Country Club Drive
Carson City, NV 89703
Phone: 775-884-3990
Fax: 775-884-2202
Web site: www.antiagingmedicine.com
E-mail: doctor@antiagingmedicine.com, NVCenter@nvbell.net

Training Date: Trained with Dr. Ayre in 2002.
Conditions treated with IPT: Dr. Shallenberger treats cancer with IPT.
Practice Focus: Bases his treatments on Bio-Energy testing, which determines energy production levels, and combines results with homeopathic medicine for a specific program to increase strength, produce energy, and kill cancer.

You guys are going to love Mike. I first met Mike about a year ago. He came into the clinic tired, emaciated, and weak. Mike had stage IV esophageal cancer, and it had all but completely worn him down.

The cancer had blocked his esophagus to the point that he could not swallow anything, even his own saliva. Mike didn't have much going for himself except a certain rugged toughness, and a lot of hope. It was my job to make certain that his hope was validated.

His doctors had placed a J-tube into Mike a few weeks before. A J-tube is a feeding tube that goes through the abdomen directly into the intestines. If it were not for this tube, Mike would probably have died before I had a chance to see him. The only way he could sustain himself was to puree food, and inject it directly into his intestines through the J-tube. As you will soon see, this J-tube ended up having a particular significance for Mike.

His doctors at the hospital where he had the tube placed were direct. They told him that his condition was terminal. The cancer had spread into his lungs, and even if they surgically removed it from the esophagus, they could not eradicate it from his lungs. The best they could do was to give him some chemotherapy, which, according to his oncologist, would at best serve to lengthen his life only a few months. At worst, it might even end it sooner. Mike asked him if there was any chance that the therapy might allow him to have the tube removed, and his doctor told him no. He was going to take that tube with him to the grave.

Mike's position looked bleak. But Mike was no stranger to bleak situations. He had been in many of them before. Having grown up as a commercial fisherman on an island in Alaska, Mike had been used to braving life-threatening storms for most of his life. So he didn't give up. Instead, he found out about the most exciting breakthrough in cancer therapy today—IPT.

Insulin Potentiation Therapy

IPT stands for Insulin Potentiation Therapy. I have explained IPT and how it works in my report on cancer, but let me review that again.

In short, IPT is simply an alternative way of giving chemotherapy. But IPT is very different from regular chemotherapy. It selectively targets the chemotherapy drugs directly to the cancer cells, while it bypasses healthy cells. Because of this, IPT is safe, and has little to no side effects.

IPT exploits the fact that cancer cells, unlike healthy cells, are not able to metabolize fat for energy. They rely completely on glucose (sugar/carbohydrates) for their energy supply. This is a weakness of cancer cells, and we can use this weakness to control them. We use the hormone insulin to do this.

When insulin is injected into a patient, it has the effect of causing the patient's blood glucose to drop. As the blood glucose drops, the patient's healthy cells simply shift over to fat metabolism. But the patient's cancer cells become seriously compromised.

Shutting down the amount of glucose that a cancer cell can have has the same effect as depriving it of oxygen. You know what it's like to hold your breath. You know you can do it for one to two minutes, but much longer than that and you will quickly die. Depriving cancer cells of glucose has the same effect. If it were possible to completely deprive them of glucose, they would die within a matter of minutes, and that would be that. Unfortunately we can't do that, as I will explain later, but we can decrease the amount of glucose by at least 60-75 percent. And this is just enough of a decrease to cause them to go into an emergency mode. It is when they are in this emergency state that they are very vulnerable to chemotherapy drugs.

Cancer cells love glucose. They can't get enough. The faster they get glucose, the faster they can grow and spread. They depend on glucose so much that unlike normal cells, they actually make and release their own insulin. Remember, insulin is the hormone that allows cells, including cancer cells, to take up glucose. By making their own insulin, cancer cells guarantee that they will always have enough glucose. Not only that but they also have another mechanism helping them get more and more glucose. I'm talking about insulin receptors.

When insulin comes into contact with a cell, it has to interact with an area on the surface of the cell called an insulin receptor. Insulin can't work to pump glucose into a cell unless it can find an insulin receptor to work through. So cancer cells are smart. Not only do they make their own insulin, they also create hundreds of times more insulin receptors for the insulin to interact with. All this is to ensure that they have enough glucose to thrive and grow.

So when the blood glucose levels start falling after the insulin injection, cancer cells start to get worried. And they start to activate and increase the number of insulin receptors. The longer they are deprived of glucose, the more they activate these receptors, and the weaker they get. It's too bad that we can't just take the blood glucose level all the way down to zero. If we could do that, every cancer cell in the body would be dead within a matter of minutes.

The reason we can't do this has to do with the brain. Unlike all of the other cells of the body, nerve cells are not able to survive on only fat, they must have some glucose. That's why it is impossible to decrease the glucose levels down to zero. We would knock off brain cells, and put the patient into a coma. So instead, here's what we do.

We give enough insulin to the patient to take his or her blood glucose level down to the point at which his brain cells start to feel the pinch. Typically, this is at a level of about 35-45 mg/dL. At this level patients will start to feel "fuzzy" or lightheaded. They may also feel weak, hungry, and flushed. The insulin dose is adjusted to keep them in this state for five to six minutes. This is enough time to cause every cancer cell in the body to panic, and open all of its glucose floodgates. Then at the right moment, the magic of IPT occurs.

That's when we then inject the chemotherapy drugs, immediately followed by an intravenous infusion of a large amount of glucose. What happens next is that as the cancer cells, now sufficiently weakened and starved for glucose, take up the glucose that they so desperately need, they also take up the chemotherapy drugs. Just like a Trojan horse, the glucose molecules carry the chemo drugs right into the heart of the cancer cells. It has been calculated that this technique causes about ten times more of the drugs to get into the cancer cells than regular chemotherapy does.

The effect of IPT is twofold. First, the cancer cells will take up much larger amounts of chemotherapy medications than they ordinarily would without the insulin application. Second, since they are in such a weakened and vulnerable state from the lack of sugar, they are much more sensitive to the toxic effects of the drugs. The result is a level of cancer cell death and growth control comparable to or even better than standard chemotherapy. But there is one very big difference.

IPT is Gentle

Because the IPT technique results in a higher concentration of the chemo-therapeutic drugs in the cancer cells, we are able to use much lower chemotherapy doses than are normally used. In general, we usually use about one-tenth of the standard dose. And this has two big advantages.

First, the lower dose means that there are little to no side effects. Our patients typically feel as good as ever—even immediately after the treatments. Second, and perhaps more importantly, because the doses are so low, IPT treatments can be used as long as they are needed without the concern of long-term toxicity to healthy cells and tissues. Unlike with conventional chemotherapy, with IPT we can keep right on using the treatments for months and even years. As long as it takes to do the job.

A Death Sentence

Mike came to see me because he learned about IPT on the Internet at www.iptforcancer.com. He carefully considered all of his options, including talking it all over with his surgeon and his oncologist, and came to the conclusion that IPT made the most sense.

When I first saw Mike, he looked pretty bad. He had not eaten or drunk anything for a month. He had lost thirty-five pounds, and was weak enough to need help walking into the examination room. I explained to him that I could not make any guarantees about how well he would respond, but I did point out one very positive thing—he had not had any conventional chemotherapy.

It's my opinion that for stage III and stage IV cancers, conventional chemotherapy is a death sentence. I can say this because my experience and that of all of the other doctors who use IPT has been the same. The only time we see full-blown remissions is in patients who have not had their immune systems wiped out with conventional chemo.

IPT will kill cancer cells, that we know. But the only chance that anyone with cancer has for a long-term remission is if, after the cancer cells are killed, the person's immune system is functioning well enough to keep the cancer from coming back. Just killing cancer cells is not enough. A real cure means having a fully active immune system.

Conventional chemotherapy poisons the immune system just as much as it poisons the cancer cells; when the cancer comes back, it comes back with a vengeance. Whereas before a patient has conventional chemotherapy, at least some immune system is working on his or her behalf; after chemotherapy, what little was there is gone or nearly gone. And in this weakened state, when the cancer comes back, there is very little left to slow it down, much less keep it controlled.

I told Mike that since he did not have conventional chemo, he still had a fighting chance. So we went to work.

"I Want That Tube!"

Like most doctors who use IPT, I integrate it with a very intensive program combining immune system enhancement, aggressive detoxification, and rejuvenation therapy. So Mike not only received his IPT treatments twice a week, he was also busy during the other days. He took an individualized program of hormones, vitamins, minerals, and herbs to build up his strength. Of course he couldn't just swallow the supplements. They had to be soaked and dissolved in water in order to be injected down his J-tube.

He also had regular immune-enhancing vaccine injections, colonics, massages, detoxifying foot baths, and intravenous infusions of massive doses of vitamin C.

For the first several weeks it was touch and go. He was so weak, and his blood counts were so low that even these simple therapies were a push for his dilapidated system. But, as I told you, Mike was tough. He didn't say much, but he received all of his treatments like clockwork, bearing pain, nausea, and weakness with great courage.

Three weeks went by and his condition seemed about the same. He asked, "When am I going to get better?" And I said, "Give it a few more weeks; at least you're not getting any worse. Your weight is holding on, and there's no evidence that the cancer is growing like it was." A week later an amazing thing happened. Mike told me that he was starting to swallow some saliva. That was an extremely encouraging sign, and because of this we decided that his IPT treatments could be decreased to once a week.

My wife, Judy, holds regular cooking classes for all of our patients. You can see her in action by going to www.video.google.com and entering her name into the search engine. When Judy gives her classes, she actually cooks the food (we have a cooking classroom in the clinic), and then has all of the attendees sample the food. I'm telling you this because at about the sixth week, Mike went to Judy's class, and Judy told me that he ate some of the food that she had prepared. I don't blame him. Judy is a great cook. It was the first food he had swallowed in almost two months! Another sign of things to come.

About one month later, Mike was eating full-time. He hadn't used his tube in weeks. And he was gaining back his weight. He was starting to look like the commercial fisherman he was before all this happened. He was driving by himself, and was essentially self-sufficient. So I asked him if he wanted me to take the J-tube out. He had two considerations. First, he wasn't looking forward to having a tube pulled out that went right into the interior of his abdomen. Second, he was afraid that the great response he was having might not last, and so he wanted to play it safe for a while longer.

That while lasted about two more months. By that time, it was apparent that he was going into a remission. He felt great, was fully functional, and was eating and drinking without difficulty. His CT scan came back indicating that the cancer in his esophagus and his lungs had receded about 75 percent. Mike wasn't looking forward to it, but he knew the time had come. I gave Mike a shot of a strong narcotic. I also injected the area around the tube with an anesthetic. And then we laid him down, and I gave a big tug on the J-tube. Out it came with a pop, and that was that.

I started to toss the tube away when Mike said, "Wait a minute, Doc. I want that thing. I'm going to wait until next year and then give it back to the doctor that told me I was going to die with it. I can't wait to see his face."

A Life Sentence

Two months after the tube incident, I sent Mike home to Alaska. I was running a little low on salmon and halibut, and I couldn't see any reason to keep him in Carson City any longer. I knew he was itching to get back to the sea. So I let him go, with the understanding that he was going to return once a month for an IPT treatment, and to deliver some fresh halibut steaks, until he was completely free of disease. He e-mailed me a few weeks later telling me about a four-hundred-pound halibut that he just hauled into his boat. The fact that he was able to do that so soon after all he had been through was just amazing to me.

In November of 2008, we repeated Mike's CT-scan. This time it showed that the cancer was "almost gone." There were still some shadows on the scan, but these could have been just scar tissue replacing the cancer that had been there. To make sure, we had a gastroenterologist put a scope down Mike's esophagus. The report?

Scar tissue, but NO CANCER. But Mike wasn't ready to have a party yet. There was still the issue of the cancer in the lungs.

To evaluate this, I ordered a PET scan. Unlike a CT scan, which cannot always tell the difference between scar tissue and cancer, a PET scan can. This is because a PET scan uses the same approach to seeing a cancer as IPT uses to killing it. In a PET scan, radioactive glucose is injected into the patient, and then the scanning device is able to see if there are any cancer cells that are taking up the glucose. A negative PET scan means no active cancer. The result? NO CANCER.

Is It Possible To Have No Cancer?

Did this mean that Mike really had no cancer anywhere? Not in my mind. You see, according to autopsy studies, everybody gets cancer. In fact, almost everybody gets more than one kind of cancer. At the age of sixty-two, I'd be willing to bet that I have at least two different cancers. When you think about it, it's only natural. Sooner or later, the longer you live, the more likely some of your cells are going to mutate. But that's not the end of the story.

The kind of cancers I'm talking about are called "occult" or "latent" cancers. That's because they can be discovered only when they are carefully looked for as part of an autopsy. In real life, these cancers don't become an issue. They are surrounded and held in check by the immune system, and they aren't able to grow more than about three-eighths of an inch. They won't grow beyond that or ever become a medical problem unless something happens that suppresses the immune system and allows them to get out of hand.

And so I can expect Mike to be free of any clinical cancer for many years to come. That's because he was not treated with conventional chemotherapy, which means his immune system is still intact. And in addition, he has improved his immune system function with the therapies that he had in the clinic, and ones that he is still doing. Here's what Mike told me in an e-mail he sent last month (January 2009):

Thank you again for all you did—I'm still getting use to being alive, kind of a strange feeling... I almost feel like I have to make something out of my life now that I had to work so hard to keep it. Things were a lot easier when I got squeezed out the first time and had no say in the matter."

In about two more months I don't think I will have to remind Mike that it will be time to take his old J-tube on over to the doctor who should be pretty surprised to see him walk in the door.

❧

CHAPTER 9

The Nevada Center

A Patient's Journey

By Michael Short—Petersburg, Alaska

In March of 2008 I was diagnosed with esophageal cancer. Several weeks later, after a needle biopsy on my lung, I learned that the cancer had metastasized. My oncologist told me the cancer was stage IV and said I had no chance of survival.

I was diagnosed at Sutter Cancer Center in Sacramento, California, which is supposed to be one of the better cancer centers in the United States. The diagnosis was not a mistake—I could see the cancer on all of the PET and CT scans, and the throat scope where it showed up in full color. In addition to the full color pictures, I was having more and more trouble swallowing.

I was told get my affairs in order because I had less than six months to live without treatment. My oncologist recommended I do chemotherapy right away. He claimed they needed to treat things aggressively and that the chemo would extend my life by a year, maybe two.

He didn't make much sense—after taking over six weeks to stage my cancer, *now* we needed to be aggressive? It felt like coming off the desktop and getting on the death march. Hurry up and die.

My friend Judy asked him where the hope was; he said there was none. I asked him about quality of life; he told me that it would be tough, but that they had some new drugs to ease the pain.

The main problem was that by the time I got the full diagnosis, my throat had completely closed off and I could no longer swallow.

I had to carry a cup around to spit in because even my own saliva wouldn't go down. I was slowly starving to death, partly from not being able to eat and partly because the cancer was burning up calories.

I was fifty years old. I had been in good shape. Prior to this I'd only been to a doctor to stitch up a few cuts so I didn't have a medical record or a primary care doc. I build remote cabins in Alaska, sometimes flying in or boating in with materials and supplies and not coming out until the cabins are done six months later. So I was strong and basically healthy. And now my life was over.

The more I thought about it, the more I wanted to know what was going to kill me. What exactly was cancer? I'd faced death many times in Alaska with bear attacks, with skiffs overturning in a storm, with freezing nights on remote beaches. It wasn't like death was a stranger. But I wanted to understand *why* cancer was going to kill me.

So we hit the books and the Internet. Judy and I read everything we could on the subject of cancer, sometimes spending sixteen to twenty hours a day sifting through information. At first it felt overwhelming. When you Google "cancer" or "cancer treatment," hundreds of thousands of sites come up. You don't know the snake oil from the good stuff. Judy was great at finding information and triaging it so I could scan through the best information quickly. I speed-read which helped a lot—I can read an entire book in a few hours if I'm motivated—and I was motivated. We made a good team. Judy said she needed to read survivor stories and made that her focus. I tried to learn the mechanics of cancer—what it is and how to cure it. Judy said all along that her prayer was that we find the right information and the right people in enough time. And before long, people I didn't even know were praying for me. I continued to research.

And I decided to get a stomach tube put in to buy me a little time and also a chemo port just in case I wanted to go with the chemo treatments. At that point I had enough information to be deeply concerned about the side effects of chemo and was not sure that I wanted to die that way. I also had learned a bit about alternative treatments and it looked like there might be a way to survive.

I had started out at 190 pounds and when I got out of the hospital in mid-April I weighed 150 pounds. Time was growing short.

I tried to talk over alternative forms of treatment with my oncologist and surgeon and they got mad, even shaking their fingers in my face and raising their voices in a stern, authoritative way, as if I was challenging them. I thought it was funny in a strange kind of way. What were they going to do—give me cancer? I finally just thanked them for their help, and Judy and I walked out.

By this time I knew that I didn't want standard chemo so I left Sutter Cancer Center for good. Judy and I had done enough research to discover that there were some people who survived stage IV cancer and went on to be completely cured—their cancer never came back. We were going through their stories, discovering what they had done. It was my best and only shot at survival.

Conventional medicine clearly had nothing for me. The doctors told me that they could do little more than extend my life for a year, maybe two, at the end of which I was expected to die. I knew it wouldn't be a pretty death—I'd watched several friends die of chemo poisoning. I considered doing nothing at all. I would have enough time to see my kids in Nebraska and then go out to the family cabin on Admiralty Island in Southeastern Alaska to die.

But I wanted to live. And that's important—vital, to surviving cancer.

Judy and I hit the books and the Internet again with a renewed drive. We consulted with people at various treatment centers and interviewed medical researchers and health care providers. We visited with people diagnosed with cancer.

We continued to follow Johanna Budwig's research using cottage cheese and flax oil, in my case blended with pure water in a Magic Bullet so I could get it through the feeding tube. That gave me some calories and some of the life-saving nutrients. Judy was juicing for us and making vegetable broths. So the stomach tube helped with the weight loss—I was dropping nearly one and a half pounds a day—and it bought me some critical time.

Within a week of leaving Sutter Cancer Center I knew the top four protocols I wanted to try. After a lot of research and a few more days, we found a doctor that would give them to me. IPT was the key criterion we were looking for in a doctor, followed by ozone, DMSO, and Vitamin C.

Our research led us to Frank Shallenberger, MD, HMD, at The Nevada Center in Carson City. He had the best of allopathic medicine, and a belief and experience in homeopathic and orthomolecular medicine. He could bring all this into the fight and find solutions to cancer that conventional medicine completely misses. And he was a maverick enough to have been called to task by the medical board. We saw this as a plus—he wasn't part of the system we'd learned to distrust.

Judy drove us over the Sierra Nevada Mountains with me slumped in the seat. I don't remember much of the drive beyond a few trees going by and high mountain passes. We walked into The Nevada Center the last week in April to see what it looked like and meet the people involved. I weighed about 134 pounds.

Dr. Shallenberger took one look at me and had me hooked up to an IV that afternoon. The appointment I'd made by Phone prior to just arriving on the scene for a tour wasn't for two more weeks, but both Dr. Shallenberger and his wife, who administers The Nevada Center, told me there was no time to lose. Good thing, I doubt if I had much more than a few weeks left.

I started the four-day-a-week treatment program, with the protocols I'd wanted, along with therapies that would detox my body and build my immune system. Besides the IVs, I took infrared saunas, ionic footbaths, colonics, and supplements. Judy continued to juice for us; everything went through the feeding tube.

In two and a half weeks I could swallow won-ton soup broth. In five weeks I could go to a buffet and get my money's worth. I continued with treatment at The Nevada Center from April 22 until mid-August.

Then in the middle of August I went to Alaska for a month to walk the beaches, fish, go deer hunting with my brothers, and visit with my parents. I needed to know I was alive, and I needed to do some of the things that for me made life worth living.

In mid-September I came down for a week of treatment and went back to Alaska for another month. There were still clams to dig and black cod to smoke. And I'd told Judy I'd take her moose hunting.

We returned to Carson City in late October and stayed for treatment until almost Christmas. On the sixteenth of December we got the results back from the PET scan and throat scope. There was no sign of cancer. It was completely gone. With that news the infusion room erupted in cheers and applause. I'm sure I smiled, but I was kind of stunned at the same time.

Unbelievable. Stage IV cancer with no hope of survival in April to completely cured by the middle of December. Eight months. Absolutely unbelievable. I still have a hard time realizing that it's true. I'd spent so much energy and time in a focused fight with cancer and now it was gone. Conventional medicine told me that this was impossible—I was condemned to die with no hope of survival. Clearly this wasn't true.

We had several friends who were fighting cancer around the same time I was diagnosed. None of them survived. I talked with them during my treatments and they told me they were happy with their doctors and conventional medicine. They carried that faith to their graves. We found that people would rather accept the certainty of death than risk a chance at life.

Dr. Shallenberger has one of the best programs that I've found for treating cancer. His treatment works, and works well, which is far more than I can say for any conventional medical treatments unless you're just the one in a thousand who survives it. I've found Dr. Shallenberger to be an honest, compassionate man who is deeply committed to his patients. He's a skilled healer. I recommend him with no reservation whatsoever. If my cancer ever comes back I won't hesitate to walk through his clinic door once again.

We had worried about the costs of cancer. And for good reason. With conventional treatment it usually costs between $350,000 and a half million dollars or more to die of cancer in this country, and that's with good insurance coverage that pays 80 percent. Cancer bankrupts people who are left to pay 20 percent of those huge amounts. We found that for about 10 percent of those costs a person could seek select alternative treatments, and get to live.

I wake up every morning with new appreciation…and in the back of my mind is the thought of how different it could have been. I realize how fortunate I was to learn about IPT and to find Dr. Shallenberger. If I had continued with conventional treatment I would probably not have survived the year and would be dying just about now. Instead I'm enjoying the sunrises over the mountains in the mornings, appreciating each day's routines, hanging out in the company of good friends, planning a new future, and having the opportunity to share what I've learned this past year.

Together, Judy and I continue to learn more about wellness, with a big emphasis on diet, nutrition, and the body's' neurology. And we keep meeting incredible people.

CHAPTER 10

IPT – Insulin Potentiation Therapy –
Vision for the Future

By David C. Korn, DDS, DO, MD (H)

Dr. Korn has twenty-seven years of Allopathic, Alternative Medicine, Natural Medicine, and Homeopathic Medical experience. He is highly trained in chelation therapy, IPT-LowDose™ chemotherapy, H2O2, Ozone and vitamin C IV. All of this special training makes Dr. Korn an expert in the treatment of the immune system.

Contact:	**David Korn, MD (H), DO, DDS**
	Medical Director of Long Life Medical, Inc.
Address:	6632 E. Baseline Rd. Ste. 101
	Mesa, AZ 85206
Phone:	480-354-6700
Fax:	480-354-6708
Web site:	http://www.longlife-medical.com
E-mail:	longlifemedical@earthlink.net

Training Date: Dr. Korn trained with Dr. Ayre in 2001

Conditions Treated with IPT: Cancer, Lyme Disease, Bacteria, Viruses, and Autoimmune Disorders.

Practice Focus: Dr. David C. Korn is the Medical Director for the newest FDA study for a vaccine for Natural Killer Cells, they are called "natural" killers because they, unlike Cytotoxic T cells, do not need to recognize a specific antigen before swinging into action. Dr. Korn questions the primary reason, "WHY" the cancer happened in the first place. The care plans for individuals are specific: IPT, Intrathecal Injections into the Tumors, "One of a kind," German Hyperthermia Beds, Stem Cells, Detoxification, Ozone/Oxybosh, Vitamin C IV, Whole Food Diet, Colonics/Enemas, Massage, Homeopathics/Biofeedback, Spiritual/Prayer if desired. Dr. Korn works with a team of experts for certain diagnostic lab and gene testing, stem cells, surgery, radiation/Tomo, or hospitalization care if needed. Dr. Korn has twenty-seven years of experience and knows what is best. Dr. Korn's philosophy is, "Where The Best Of All Medical Worlds Come Together."

In 2001, I was fortunate to have participated in one of the first IPT courses available to Americans. It was taught at the American Oxidative Medicine Association. Dr. Donato Garcia III taught the class, along with Dr. Steven Ayre. I found the course absolutely intriguing, but I wanted to learn more, so I traveled to Chicago to study directly with Dr. Stephen Ayre, one-on-one.

Following my training, I began using IPT in my practice, Longlife Medical in Mesa, Arizona (www.longlife-medical.com), and became certified in IPT low-dose chemotherapy. I envisioned many potential uses for IPT; therefore, I brought Dr. Ayre to Arizona, where he taught a two-day course to our physicians.

Since I first received training, I've given several hundred IPT treatments to my patients, and the results have been remarkable! As background for the amazing case I will be sharing with you, here is a brief history of Insulin Potentiation Therapy, or IPT.

Insulin was discovered in 1921, and its use in diabetic patients first occurred in 1922. It was one of the first wonder drugs.

IPT has been used for three generations or sixty-eight to seventy years. The first physician to use it was Dr. Donato Garcia I, who was licensed in Mexico. Dr. Garcia's study and use of IPT originated from his personal experience with IPT.

In Mexico, insulin was authorized for use for diabetes and wasting disease. Dr. Garcia was suffering from wasting disease, and therefore, decided to use the treatment himself. Wasting disease occurs when nutrients are not absorbed for use by the body.

The foods Dr. Garcia ate could not parlay into weight gain. So, Dr. Garcia self-administered shots of insulin. Immediately afterward he noticed that he became ravenous for food. He repeated the "treatments" several times, and eventually, was able to put on weight.

He was ultimately able to defeat the wasting disease through his use of IPT. Dr. Garcia determined that his successful results with weight gain must have been due to potentiation of absorption. So he thought IPT might also be helpful when using other drugs to potentiate the effects. Therefore, he began utilizing insulin along with other therapies for better results in his patients.

Mechanisms for IPT to Potentiate Low-Dose Chemotherapy

Insulin potentiation of chemotherapy relates to the anatomic and physiologic fact that cancer cells have twelve to sixteen times the insulin and IGF1 receptor sites that normal cells do. The metabolism of a cancer cell requires twelve to sixteen times the IGF1, which is a type of insulin growth factor hormone. The insulin receptor of any cell is the site where the insulin fits and opens the door to the interior of the cell. Therefore, when you treat a cancer cell by lowering the blood glucose level, you somehow open twelve to sixteen times the number of doors to the interior of the cancer cell.

Glucose must enter the cell's interior with the assistance of insulin. It has to go through the cell membrane, which selectively allows various substances in and out of the cell. Next, the glucose has to permeate the nuclear membrane and finally permeate the mitochondrial membrane. The mitochondria are the energy factories of every living cell.

In order to survive, the mitochondria of every cell produce ATP (adenosine triphosphate), and our bodies have to have it to function.

Cancer cells also need glucose and actually thrive on it. Due to the large number of insulin receptor sites, the cancer cells are able to absorb the insulin/glucose quite readily. All the glucose that cancer cells can absorb, even if you don't eat much, is going to steal every molecule of sugar, and thereby steal your energy. This ravenous hunger of the cancer cells starves the other cells of the body of insulin/ glucose, thereby lowering the amount of ATP created by the healthy cells. In this way, cancer cells create an energy deficit, thereby lowering our energy level.

Linus Pauling proved long ago with X-ray refraction that hormones are released by an endocrine gland. The hormone then goes into the bloodstream to the receptor sites on the cells of different organs. Dr. Pauling demonstrated that chemicals and hormones do not exist in a textbook flat plane, but in Tinker toy design, with projections sticking out in various directions.

The hormones must bind to the receptor sites before any hormonal reaction can occur. The desired reaction cannot occur unless it fits exactly with the receptor site. This is called stereo chemical receptor specificity. So, such specificity is required at each receptor site to allow the reaction to proceed.

IPT lowers the blood sugar level to the lowest therapeutic point of hypoglycemia in patients. This is sometimes referred to as "the moment of truth." This is accomplished with Humalog at .4 units per kilogram of body weight. The Humalog brings the blood glucose level down to about 30, which is hypoglycemia.

Dr. Garcia showed that there would be enhanced absorption of everything at the maximum hypoglycemic measurement. At this point, a dose of chemotherapy, that is 10 to 20 percent of the standard dose, is administered intravenously. This is why IPT low-dose chemotherapy is called a "gentle" cancer therapy.

In this hypoglycemic state, the cancer cells are starving for additional glucose, and the insulin allows the chemotherapy drug to enter the cancer cells more easily. IPT works in this way—1 plus 1 doesn't equal 2; due to potentiation, it equals 2.75 or 3. The IPT allows another drug to be absorbed more readily and the beneficial effects are increased dramatically. IPT improves the effects of any given drug through working together with the insulin during the process of absorption.

With IPT, you can give a much lower dose of the chemotherapy drug, and it is uniquely attracted to the cancer cells. And the drug will be maximally absorbed at the lowest-tolerable hypoglycemic level.

IPT LowDose chemotherapy allows a greater effect on the cancer cells, and there are other potentiators, as well, that increase the effects of low-dose chemotherapy. The other potentiators are DMSO (dimethyl sulfoxide), hyperthermia, electro chemotherapy and oxidative therapy.

IPT LowDose chemotherapy helps prevent the awful side effects of high-dose chemotherapy, such as hair loss and mouth ulcerations.

The primary focus of this book is on the modality Insulin Potentiation Targeted LowDose™ Chemotherapy (IPTLD™) / Insulin Potentiation Therapy (IPT) for treatment of cancer. However, the following additional applications are presented to demonstrate the broad healing potential IPT/IPTLD™ offers the medical community and patients. Stay tuned for our upcoming book on IPTLD™ for Chronic Disease.

Lyme Disease (Borreliosis)

Lyme disease, or borreliosis, is caused by a virulent, intracellular bacterium called Borrelia burgdorferi (Bb). The majority of cases are not appropriately diagnosed in the acute stage of disease, and therefore, most patients present with embedded infections that require lengthy treatment. Standard recommendations for short-term antibiotic therapy are not working in chronic cases and patients relapse frequently.

Therefore, clinicians have tried combination therapies and pulsing to improve outcome for borreliosis patients. Recent work that has discovered biofilms and the ability of this intracellular pathogen to evade the immune system is helping to improve clinical outcome. However, clinicians face intense opposition from those who promote the short-term antibiotic regimen. This opposition has caused a great rift between physicians. Unfortunately patients ultimately land in the middle of the rift which often results on unresolved chronic infection.

When Dr. Garcia treated brain infections using IPT, he determined that the insulin and other drug therapies were able to cross the blood brain barrier (BBB). Dr. Garcia's early results also showed that insulin, in combination with the treatment drug, got past the BBB, into the brain.

In my practice, I will be exploring the use of IPT with one of the very important diseases that I have been treating, Lyme disease. Bb does invade the brain causing severe cognitive impairment; therefore, it is crucial for any therapy for borreliosis to be able to cross the BBB.

Biofilms in Chronic Infection

Clinicians who treat borreliosis are having difficulty in resolving the relapses associated with chronic Borrelia infection. Borrelia burgdorferi biofilms play a significant role in the pathogen's resistance to antibiotics.

Recently, I read research by Dr. E. Peter Greenberg of the University of Washington in Seattle, in which he studied pseudomonas aeruginosa biofilms. He applied gentamicin to pseudomonas aeruginosa in a petri dish. Gentamicin is a powerful antibiotic that can damage the ears and kidneys, if not used carefully by the practitioner. However, the gentamicin failed to kill the pseudomonas.

Next, Dr. Greenberg added EDTA (ethylenediaminetetraacetic acid), a biofilm buster, in the petri dish and added the gentamicin a second time. Sure enough, the gentamicin killed every bug in the dish. He thereby deduced that the pathogen had a biofilm.

Following that, Dr. Greenberg began the experiment anew, but this time he added magnesium to the petri dish. This result showed that the gentamicin was ineffective against the biofilm. Dr. Greenberg deduced that magnesium strengthened the biofilm, and is therefore, contraindicated for pseudomonas aeruginosa infection.

In addition to Dr. Greenberg's research on biofilms, two Lyme disease researchers have studied Borrelia burgdorferi biofilms. It has been theorized that magnesium and arginine may be contraindicated for Lyme disease. Based upon this information, we are using IV chelation with EDTA to bust open the Bb biofilms, and then we follow it with our current treatment protocol for borreliosis.

Scleroderma and Lyme Disease

Traditionally, scleroderma is a dreadful rheumatologic disorder, in which the covering of organs and the skin of our outer body begin to "clamp down" on the organs and joints. This is due to hardening of the epithelial cells, and causes crippling due to the inability to move muscles and bones through restriction of the skin and mucosa. The hands can become clawed due to hardening of the skin and loss of elasticity. Eventually, the heart muscle is unable to contract and expand due to tightening of the pericardium. This constriction limits the heart's excursion.

Scleroderma is one of over three hundred diseases that arise from borreliosis (Lyme disease). It is not widely known by rheumatologists that scleroderma is caused by Lyme disease infection, but it is documented in the literature. Scleroderma can also be caused by other infections in the human body.

Scleroderma is an uncommon and horrible disease that does not have a good prognosis. I have found that scleroderma, rheumatoid arthritis, and other rheumatoid disorders are mostly from Borrelia infection. It is my belief, after treating and supervising the treatment of approximately one thousand patients with borreliosis, that most of the autoimmune disorders that rheumatologists treat are, in fact, caused by an infection, and Borrelia is most often the infectious etiology.

Case History

One of the borreliosis (Lyme) patients I treated has been well for so long, as compared with my other Lyme patients, that I think the difference is due to the IPT I administered to her. Mrs. F was a lady who traveled from Mexico to Arizona for treatment, because she had heard that I used IPT.

She presented to my office with a serious case of scleroderma that her rheumatologist had been treating. The prognosis for Mrs. F was not favorable. However, I suspected that the scleroderma was caused by an infection. Due to the fact that she had joint, muscle and bone pain, sleep disturbance, concentration deficits, and memory loss, I had a hunch that it might be Borrelia burgdorferi.

I had read in a newsletter that IPT was used in a case of scleroderma with good results, so I considered the possible treatments and thought that using IPT with IV antibiotic might be the way to go. In this way, IPT would have the ability to potentiate the effect of the antibiotic.

At the time, I had diagnosed only two other cases of borreliosis, a female patient and me, and I was just beginning to get a handle on this infection.

I told Mrs. F and her family that I would treat her scleroderma. So, I administered IPT and IV antibiotic, and we noted a good deal of improvement. However, she relapsed three weeks later and came back to see me.

Therefore, we administered one more IPT treatment, and after we got Mrs. F's glucose to the lowest tolerable hypoglycemic level once more, we pushed her IV antibiotics. After again improving after this additional treatment, she relapsed once more, and it was then that I told Mrs. F and her family that I thought she had Lyme disease.

You see, one push of antibiotic is not going to cure anyone with a serious case of borreliosis. To make a dent in an embedded Borrelia infection, you must begin with eight weeks of IV antibiotics three times per day. So, I told Mrs. F and her family that, because I thought she might have Borreliosis, I would like to do a blood test for confirmation.

I sent Mrs. F's blood to the lab, but she was seronegative for Bb. I knew that her clinical diagnosis was positive though. Therefore, when her entire family was gathered in my small treatment room to hear the results, it took all the courage I could muster to tell them her test had come back negative.

You see, they were all so excited to hear whether their wife and mother had a different diagnosis—a diagnosis that would give them hope for her survival. So, when I had to tell them that the serology was negative, it was very difficult.

I looked them squarely in the eyes, and I sadly said that her Western blot tests were negative for Lyme. Now, at the time, Mrs. F had a number of indeterminate bands on her test, and because I did not have the extensive experience in reading Lyme tests, as I do now after a thousand patients, I was unable to see that there were some indications that she could have been positive.

Now, I can recognize such a test result that indicates an immune system that is too weak to respond to the antigenic provocation of the Borrelia kilodalton bands. In retrospect, I now know that there was a need to repeat the testing in three to four weeks following antibiotic treatment.

The family dejectedly looked me in the eyes and asked me, "What now, Doctor?" And I told them that I thought that Mrs. F did indeed have Lyme disease and that the test was a false negative. I explained the difficulty with Bb test results, and I told them I would treat the Lyme disease despite the negative test result. I asked them, "What do you have to lose?" And they agreed.

So, I treated Mrs. F with IV antibiotics for Lyme disease for an additional eight weeks, and to this day, she responded better than any of my other Lyme patients. What amazes me the most is that Mrs. F recovered from the scleroderma. For the past six years, she relapsed only once for a very short period and has remained well ever since.

When she returned to her rheumatologist for testing, her respiratory functions at a university hospital had improved threefold on each test. She no longer needed the dangerous lung drug that the rheumatologist had prescribed. Secondly, her heart trouble had resolved. And thirdly, her hands were returning to normal and were no longer clawed. She was able to stop taking all the drugs the rheumatologist had prescribed. She was taking only various nutrients that I had suggested.

The rheumatologist became so enraged over the fact that Mrs. F was cured, that he threw his pen on his desk in front of the family and said, "I tell you I am the world's authority on scleroderma, and she is going to die from this disease!" That was a horrible thing to say to someone who was markedly improved. However, it appears that he was jealous and angry that <u>he</u> wasn't able to cure her.

Vision of Health

I have come to the conclusion that IPT may be one of the most important treatments that we're overlooking when it comes to a worldwide epidemic of chronic infections. Applying IPT with antimicrobial and antiviral therapy, Vitamin C IV, UVBI, oxygen therapy, a high-nutrient diet, fasting and juicing, acupuncture, muscle testing, enzymes, PH balancing, and detoxification should provide our patients with all the tools they need to recover from pathogen overload.

I will continue to provide updates as they occur and post them on my Web site at www.longlife-medical.com.

With Insulin Potentiation Therapy, the possibilities are endless, and the vision of being able to restore balance to bodies that have been struggling for so long is truly joyous!

CHAPTER 11
How to Become a Certified IPT/IPTLD™ Physician

There are certain requirements to be met and guidelines to follow in order to become certified as an IPTLD™ Physician. These are some of the basic requirements:

- Physician must be licensed as either an MD or DO in the jurisdiction in which he or she practices

- Physician must have at least five years' experience as a practicing MD or DO

- Physician must pay the appropriate fees to the Instructor (certified by The Best Answer for Cancer Foundation℠ Board of Directors) and complete a five-day training session with a certified IPT instructor

- Physician must establish membership with the International Organization of IPT Physicians by contacting Rebecca@iptforcancer.com and paying the appropriate fees.

- Physician must pass a written, online test on administering the therapy

- Physician must maintain his or her membership in the International Organization of IPT Physicians (IOIP) in good standing

To receive an **IPT Training Application, a list of all certified IPT Instructors**, and more information on **IOIP Membership Benefits,** please e-mail Rebecca Ayre at: <u>rebecca@elkabest.org</u>

Appendix

A. Frequently Asked Questions

B. Directory of IPTLD™ Physicians

C. Resources: Web Sites, Books, and Articles

D. History of IPTLD™

E. IPTLD™ Treatment at a Glance

F. Glossary

APPENDIX A

Frequently Asked Questions

What is Insulin Potentiation Targeted LowDose™ (IPTLD™)?*[1]

IPT is the historic name for a procedure discovered by Donato Perez Garcia, MD, in 1929 that allowed the specific targeting of diseased cells by traditional drugs, thus requiring a fractionated dose of the drugs.

It was first used on cancer in 1946. IPT as a therapy for cancer is a procedure for administering conventional FDA-approved chemotherapeutic drugs *in fractionated doses directly to the cancer* cells instead of the whole body. It is a process that turns cancer cells' characteristic ability to live against themselves. Insulin Potentiation Targeted LowDose™ (IPTLD™) is the current name (researched and assigned in 2006 by The Best Answer for Cancer Foundation℠ to more accurately describe the therapy) for that same procedure. Only the name has changed; the procedure is the same.

Why is IPTLD™ needed?

Over time conventional chemotherapy dosages may so compromise the patient's blood counts, immune system, and organ function as to preclude further treatment or even cause organ damage resulting in the patient's death. Additionally, there are some patients whose

---

1   *The name IPT (Insulin Potentiation Therapy) has recently been changed to IPTLD™ (Insulin Potentiation Targeted LowDose™). **IPTLD™** is the current name (researched, reserved, and assigned in 2006 by Annie Brandt and the board of The Best Answer for Cancer FoundationSM to more accurately describe the therapy) for that same procedure. Only the name has changed to better represent the technique; the therapy remains the same. Throughout this book, you will see both names. Please consider them synonymous.

bodies and/or immune systems could not withstand the rigors of conventional chemotherapy.

IPTLD™ gives patients the power of chemo to the cancer cells only, not to the healthy cells. IPTLD™™ eliminates the "lesser of two evils" decision all cancer patients face when diagnosed. Patients thrive as they experience a gentle and effective answer to cancer. IPTLD™ is truly an example of the goal to "First Do No Harm."

What are the dangers of conventional chemotherapy?

Cancer cells are voracious in fighting for the life-sustaining glucose found in the blood stream. With sixteen times the number of insulin receptors of a healthy cell, cancer cells steal any and all essential nutrients from good cells. This is why, in advanced stages of this disease, a tumor continues to grow while the patient becomes emaciated and simply wastes away. Added to this, because of membrane protection from toxins, standard administered chemotherapy must be in large enough quantities to force penetration of cell walls. This results in the indiscriminate penetration and killing of both healthy and cancerous cells as well as most frequently leaving the patient with fever, nausea, vomiting, hair loss, diminished quality of life.

To put it in simple terms, conventional chemotherapy: damages the immune system and vital body organs; destroys the P53 tumor suppressor gene; distorts the DNA of healthy cells, making them precancerous; causes cancer to build immunities to the chemos, thus making cancer stronger; and usually causes side-effects that significantly lessen quality-of-life.

How does IPTLD™ work?

IPTLD™ uses insulin to stimulate division in cancer cells. Remember, cancer cells have sixteen times the number of insulin receptors than healthy cells. Chemotherapy penetrates better when cells are dividing. The insulin causes a lowering of the blood sugar to the point that the healthy cells are no longer actively involved, but the cancer cells are voraciously active. This is the "therapeutic moment" and the time at which the chemo is delivered *to the cancer cells*.

Because of this targeted action, IPTLD™ uses only 10–15 percent of conventional drug doses and the procedure affects only the cancer while leaving normal cells strong and healthy. This means that patients continue to thrive, maintain their lifestyle, and feel vital while the cancer is eradicated. Thriving W<u>hile</u> Surviving^{SM}.

What are the benefits of IPTLD™?

- IPTLD™ can be very tough against tumors while being very gentle for the patient who continues to live a normal, vital lifestyle while being treated. Patients Thrive while they Survive.

- If there is a chemotherapy drug that works against a particular type of tumor, it is likely to work better with IPTLD™

- Gentle treatment may preclude the need for surgery or radiation.

- Treatment costs are significantly less than the conventional procedure.

What cancers respond to IPTLD™?

IPTLD™ has been reported to work especially well for breast, prostate, lung, colon, and stomach cancers; lymphoma; and melanoma. There are also reports of IPTLD™ bringing responses and remissions to patients with some very difficult cancers, including pancreatic, ovarian, and renal cell cancers. Other cancers successfully treated are blood, bone, cervical, esophageal, lip, mouth, neck, small intestines, testicular, throat, thyroid, uterine, and vaginal.

APPENDIX B

Directory of IPT/IPTLD™ Certified Physicians

*NOTE: Doctors must Recertify with The Best Answer for Cancer Foundation[SM] Board of Directors on a regular basis to be considered a certified IPT/IPTLD™ physician. Please check the Web site www. IPTforcancer.com or www.IPTLD.com to ensure that the doctors listed below are still active and certified physicians, which is indicated by a current directory listing on the Web site.

AUSTRALIA

Krishnan, MD, Chittoor
Coming Soon...
E-mail: chittoor1936@yahoo.co.in
Training Date: Dr. Krishnan trained with Dr. Kroiss in May 2008.

AUSTRIA

Vienna
Kroiss, MD, Thomas
Kroiss Cancer Center

Address: Speisingerstrasse 187
             Vienna A-1230

Phone: +43-1-9825767
Fax: +43-1-9826992
Web site: http://kroisscancercenter.com
E-mail: kroiss@dr-kroiss.at

Training Date: 2003 with Dr. Perez-Garcia; Instructor 2007.
Conditions treated with IPT: Dr. Kroiss uses IPT to treat cancer.

Practice Focus: Dr. Kroiss focuses on treating the underlying causes of cancer without harming the well-being of the patient.

GERMANY

Aschau
Baltin, MD, Hartmut
Dr. Med. Hartmut Baltin

Address: Zellerhorn Strasse 3
        Aschau D-83229

Phone: +49-8052-90580
Fax: +49-8052-905817
Web site: www.dr-baltin.de
E-mail: mail@dr-baltin.de

Training Date: 2003 with Dr. Perez Garcia.
Conditions treated with IPT: Dr. Baltin uses IPT to treat cancer.
Practice Focus: Dr. Baltin uses IPT with nontoxic, plant-derived substances with known tumor-killing capabilities (mistletoe, ukrain, carnivora) for cancer care.

Munich
Perticevic-Riedl, MD, Desanka
Praxis Petricevic-Riedl

Address: Gabelgererstrasse 11
        Munich D-80333

Phone: +49-89-28779313
Web site: www.Praxis-Riedl.de
E-mail: desanka@t-online.de

Training Date: 2003 with Dr. Perez Garcia. Instructor in 2006
Conditions treated with IPT: Dr. Petricevic–Riedl treats cancer and other conditions with IPT.
Practice Focus: Integrates the complementary and homeopathic with the mainstream to treat chronic pain and other degenerative diseases. Offers galvanotherapy and other treatments.

Saarbrücken
Hürtgen, MD, Geoffrey Pascal
Privatfachärztliche Praxis für Biologische Medizin

Address: Dudweilerstraße 24
Saarbrücken D-66111

Phone: +49 - 681—95 81 29 50
Fax: + 49—681—95 81 29 51
Web site: http://www.insulin-potenzierungs-therapie.de
E-mail: Dr-Huertgen@gmx.de

Training Date: 2008 with Dr. Kroiss.
Conditions treated with IPT: Dr. Hurtgen treats cancer and other conditions with IPT.
Practice Focus: Biological medicine for children and adults with chronic and oncological illnesses.

INDIA

Bangalore
Donki, MD, Jagadish
Jagadish G. Donki, MD

Address: 1187 5th Block 12th Main Road
Dhobi Ghat, Rajajinagar, Bangalore 5600010

Phone: 0091-80-21354649
Fax: 0091-80-21354649
Mobile: 0091-80-9845917230
E-mail: docjag2001@yahoo.com

Training Date: Trained with Dr. George in 2004.
Conditions treated with IPT: Dr. Donki treats cancer with IPT.
Practice Focus: Dr. Donki was the first physician in India to be trained in IPT.

MEXICO

Tijuana
Garcia, MD, Donato Perez
Donato Perez Garcia, MD

Address: Paseo de los Hereos
10999-807 Zona Urbana Rio
Tijuana, BC

Phone: +52 664-686-5473
Fax: +52 664-635-1886
Web site: www.donatoperezgarcia.com
E-mail: drrdonato3@yahoo.com

Training Date: Trained with Dr. Perez Garcia y Bellon in 1983. He is a certified Instructor.
Conditions treated with IPT: Dr. Perez Garcia uses IPT for cancer.
Practice Focus: Dr. Perez specializes solely in IPT and the well-being of his patients during the treatment.

Mexico D.F.
Herrera Flor, MD, Manuel J.
Ozonocenter Mexico

Address: Av. Monterrey No. 150 Desp 308 Col Roma Delg.
Cuautemoc Mexico, D.F.

Phone: (55) 57-15-51-07, (55) 55-64-50-54
Fax: (55) 82-83-19-66
Web site: http://www.ozonocentermexico.com
E-mail: ozonocentermexico@yahoo.com.mx

Training Date: 2003.
Conditions treated with IPT: Dr. Herrera uses IPT for cancer and other conditions.
Practice Focus: We continuously improve our IPT practice through implementation of quality systems to provide added value to our patients.

SOUTH AFRICA

Centurion
Pretorius, MD, Eugene
Centre for Advanced Medicine and Anti-Aging

Address: 75 Lyttleton Rd. Club View
Centurion 0157

Phone: +27 72-444-9959
Fax: +27 12-654-7587
E-mail: advancemedsa@yahoo.com
Web site: www.advancemedsa.com

Training Date: 2005 with Dr. Perez Garcia.
Conditions Treated with IPT: Dr. Pretorius treats cancer with IPT.
Practice Focus: Dr. Pretorius aims to treat the whole patient, focus on causes of disease, and improve immunity for numerous ailments. In addition to IPT, he uses dendritic cell therapy.

Parys
Lindeque, MD, Gerrie
Dr. Gerrie Lindeque, LMCC

Address: Buitenstreet 24
Parys 9585

Phone: +56-817-6217
Fax: +56-817-6935
E-mail: drg@lantic.net

SPAIN

Málaga
Peral, MD, Eudoxia Lopez
Clinica Medico

Address: Plaza Solidaridad 7 1 B, 29002 Málaga Spain

Phone: 034 952368146
E-mail: doxia58@yahoo.es
Conditions Treated with IPT: Dr. Peral treats cancer with IPT.

UNITED STATES
Alaska

<u>Anchorage</u>
Ellenburg, ND, MD (H), Michael J.
Comprehensive Medicine, LLC

Address: 615 East 82nd Avenue, Ste. 300
Anchorage, AK 99518

Phone: 907-344-7775
Fax: 907-522-3114
Web site: www.comprehensivemedicine.net
E-mail: mellenburg@acsalaska.net

Training Date: 2006 with Sean Devlin, MD.
Conditions treated with IPT: Dr. Ellenburg treats cancer with IPT.
Practice Focus: Dr. Ellenburg follows a comprehensive cancer treatment program, utilizing naturopathy, nutritional counseling, and bio-identical hormone treatment.

<u>Soldotna</u>
Thompson, MD, Robert

Address: 188 West Marydale Ave   **and**
6251 Tuttle Place
Soldotna, AK 99669
Anchorage, AK 99507

Phone: 907-260-6914 (Soldotna) **and** 907-565-4609 (Anchorage)
Fax: 907-260-6924
Web site: http://www.drt-obgyn.com/
E-mail: drtobgyn@hotmail.com

Training Date: 2007 with Dr. Perez Garcia.
Conditions treated with IPT: Contact office directly for information.
Practice Focus: In addition to providing IPT, Dr. Thompson is a Certified Reproductive Surgeon and an Advanced Pelviscopic Surgeon, and an In Vitro Consultant for the University of Washington. His office provides advanced, minimally invasive surgery, avoiding abdominal incisions and ensuring quicker recovery.

Arizona

Mesa
Korn, MD(H), DO, DDS, David
Long Life Medical, Inc.

Address: 6632 E. Baseline Rd. Ste. 101
Mesa, AZ 85206

Phone: 480-354-6700
Fax: 480-354-6708
Web site: http://www.longlife-medical.com
E-mail: longlifemedical@earthlink.net

Training Date: Dr. Korn trained with Dr. Ayre in 2001.
Conditions Treated with IPT: Cancer, Lyme Disease.
Practice Focus: Dr. David C. Korn is the Medical Director for the newest FDA study for a vaccine for natural killer cells, they are called "natural" killers because they, unlike cytotoxic T cells, do not need to recognize a specific antigen before swinging into action. Dr. Korn questions the primary reason, "WHY" the cancer happened in the first place. The care plans for individuals are specific: IPT, intrathecal injections into the tumors, "one of a kind," German hyperthermia beds, stem cells, detoxification, ozone/oxybosh, vitamin C IV, whole food diet, colonics/enemas, massage, homeopathics/biofeedback, and spiritual/prayer if desired. Dr. Korn works with a team of experts for certain diagnostic lab and gene testing, stem cells, surgery, radiation/Tomo, or hospitalization care if needed. Dr. Korn has twenty-seven years of experience and knows what is best. Dr. Korn's philosophy is, " Where The Best Of All Medical Worlds Come Together."
License/Certifications: DO, 1977, General Medicine and Surgery, Chicago College of Osteopathic Medicine, MD (H), 1999 Homeopathic Medical Doctor, Arizona Homeopathic Board,
DDS, 1969, Oral Pathology and Cancer, West Virginia University of Dentistry.
Associations/Societies: Sir, Dr. David C. Korn is a Certified Sovereign Medical Order Of The Knights Hospitaller Saint John Of Jerusalem, Knight of Honor Chevalier, American Medical Association, Osteopathic Medical Association, Arizona Homeopathic Medical Association, Lyme Education Awareness Program, American Cancer Society,

International Lyme Awareness Association, Elka Best Foundation, IPT, and, Fullness of Life, Stem Cells – Celebration.

Lodi, MD, Thomas
An Oasis of Healing

Address: 210 N. Center Street, Ste 102
Mesa, AZ 85201

Phone: 480-834-5414
Fax: 480-834-5418
Web site: www.anoasisofhealing.com
E-mail: info@anoasisofhealing

Training Date: Trained with Dr. Perez Garcia in 2002 and is a certified Instructor.
Conditions Treated with IPT: Dr. Lodi uses IPT to treat cancer.
Practice Focus: Teaching the patient how to stop the cancer, treat the cancer itself, and enhance the immune system through nutrition and detoxification.

Schwengel, DO, MD (H), Charles
Rhythm of Life Integrative Cancer Center

Address: 1215 E. Brown Road, Ste 2
Mesa, AZ 85203

Phone: 877-668-1448
Fax:
Web site: www.RhythmofLife.com
E-mail: info@RhythmofLife.com

Training Date: Trained with Dr. Perez Garcia in 2005.
Conditions Treated with IPT: Dr. Schwengel uses IPT to treat cancer.
Practice Focus: Integration of traditional and complementary therapies with nutritional and emotional support for cancer care. Has a Nationally Certified Massage Therapist on staff.

Phoenix
George, DO, MD (H), Frank
EuroMed LLC

Address: 34975 N. North Valley Pkwy., Unit 138
Phoenix, AZ 85086

Phone: 602-404-0400
Fax: 602-404-0403
Web site: http://www.euro-med.us/
E-mail: info@euro-med.us

Training : Dr. George trained in 2000 with Dr. Perez Garcia and is a certified instructor.
Conditions treated with IPT: EuroMed treats cancer and other diseases with IPT.
Practice Focus: EuroMed offers integrative healing therapies from all over the world for supporting the detoxification of the body, boosting of the immune system, and aiding in the treatment of cancer and other chronic diseases.

California

Oceanside (San Diego area)
Breitman, MD, Les
Winkler, MD, Juergen
Alternative Cancer Treatment Center of Southern California

Address: 2204 El Camino Real, Ste 104
Oceanside, CA 92054

Phone: 760-439-9955
Fax: 760-439-6755
Web site: www.ipthealing.com
E-mail: info@ipthealing.com

Training Date: Both doctors trained with Dr. Perez Garcia. Dr. Breitman trained in 2002 and is a certified Instructor; Dr. Winkler trained in 2005.
Conditions treated with IPT: They treat cancer with IPT.
Practice Focus: The focus is on IPT and the overall well-being of the patient. They also offers hormone therapies.

Santa Rosa
Rowen, MD, Robert

Address: P.O. Box 817
Santa Rosa, CA 95403

Phone: 707-578-7787
Fax: 707-578-7788
E-mail: doc@doctorrowen.com
Web site: http://www.secondopinionnewsletter.com

Training Date: Trained with Dr. Perez Garcia in 2000
Conditions treated with IPT: Dr. Rowen is a consultant for the Foundation in IPT.

Upland
Zuniga, MD, L.
Foothill Medical Clinic

Address: 954 W Foothill Blvd, #B
Upland, CA 91786

Phone: 909-985-8230

Training Date: Trained with Dr. Perez Garcia in 2003

Florida

Sunny Isles
Dayton, MD, DO, Martin
Dayton Medical Center

Address: 18600 Collins Avenue
Sunny Isles, FL 33160

Phone: 305-931-8484
Fax: 305-936-1849
Web site: www.daytonmedical.com
E-mail: mddomddo@pol.net

Training Date: Trained with Dr. Perez Garcia in 2001.
Conditions Treated with IPT: Dr. Dayton treats cancer with IPT.
Practice Focus: The focus is on optimizing health span in people of all ages with any ailment, combining remedial and proactive treatments, both conventional and alternative.

Illinois

Burr Ridge (Chicago area)
Ayre, MD, Steven G.
Malik, DO, Ather A.
Contemporary Medicine

Address: 322 Burr Ridge Pkwy
Burr Ridge, IL 60527

Phone: 630-321-9010
Fax: 630-321-9018
Web site:www.contemporarymedicine.net
E-mail: info@contemporarymedicine.net

Training Date: Dr. Ayre trained with Dr. Perez Garcia y Bellon in 1976 and again with Dr. Perez Garcia in 1997. He is a certified Instructor.
Conditions treated with IPT: Dr. Ayre uses IPT to treat cancer.
Practice Focus: Offers comprehensive cancer care (IPT, nutritional biochemistry, and mind/body medicine) with a kinder and gentler approach.

Indiana

Indianapolis
Guyer, MD, Dale
Advanced Medical Center and Spa

Address: 836 East 86th St.
Indianapolis, IN 46240

Phone: 317-580-9355
Fax: 317-580-9342

Web site: www.daleguyermd.com
E-mail: drguyer@insightbb.com

Training Date: Trained with Dr. Ayre in 2001.
Conditions treated with IPT: Dr. Guyer uses IPT to treat other conditions.
Practice Focus: A blended approach to health and wellness that focuses on the natural. Offers noninvasive treatments for overall well-being with nutritional support.

Michigan

Ann Arbor
Kabisch, DO, Thomas

Address: 2330 E. Stadium Suite 2
　　　　　Ann Arbor, MI 48104

Phone: 734-971-5483
Fax: 734-971-7585
E-mail: DrKabisch@naturalmedical.org

Training Date: Dr. Kabish trained with Dr. Ayre in 2002.
Conditions treated with IPT: cancer.
Practice Focus: Dr. Kabsich applies integrative medical techniques and treatments for a variety of conditions and disorders including autism, cancer, substance abuse, pain management, and muscular skeletal manipulations.

New Mexico

Santa Fe
Fitzpatrick, MD, Hennie
Integrated Health Medical Center

Address: 1532 A Cerrillos Rd.
　　　　　Santa Fe, NM 87505

Phone: 505-982-3936
E-mail: henniefitzpatrick@gmail.com

Training Date: Trained with Dr. George in 2004.

Conditions treated with IPT: Dr. Fitzpatrick treats cancer and other diseases with IPT.

Practice Focus: Strengthening and rebuilding the body through a combination of treatments based on bio-dentistry, nutritional analysis, and deep detox.

Nevada

Carson City
Shallenberger, MD, HMD, Frank
The Nevada Center

Address: 1231 Country Club Drive
Carson City, NV 89703

Phone: 775-884-3990
Fax: 775-884-2202
Web site: www.antiagingmedicine.com
E-mail: doctoro3@alpine.net, doctor@antiagingmedicine.com

Training Date: Trained with Dr. Ayre in 2002.
Conditions treated with IPT: Dr. Shallenberger treats cancer with IPT.

Practice Focus: Bases his treatments on bio-energy testing, which determines energy production levels and combines results with homeopathic medicine for a specific program to increase strength, produce energy, and kill cancer.

New York

Glen Cove
Linchitz, MD, Richard
Linchitz Medical Wellness PLLC

Address: 70 Glen Street, Ste 240
Glen Cove, NY 11542

Phone: 516-759-4200
Fax: 516-759-7600
Web site: http://linchitzwellness.com

E-mail: rlinchitz@msn.com

Training Date: Trained in 2005 with Dr. Perez Garcia.
Conditions treated with IPT: Dr. Linchitz uses IPT to treat cancer.
Practice Focus: Performs chemo-sensitivity testing along with nutritional counseling, detoxification, and energy medicine for a personal patient program.

Stony Brook
Flader, MD, William
Natural Health Alternatives

Address: 100 North Country Road
Stony Brook, NY 11733

Phone: 631-941-3137
Fax: 631-689-2994
Cell: 631-707-0043
E-mail: drflader@yahoo.com

Web site: http://ipt-health.com
Training Date: trained with Dr. Ayre in December 2007.
Conditions Treated with IPT: Dr. Flader uses IPT for cancer and other conditions.
Practice Focus: NHA, located in Suffolk County, Long Island, New York, is a holistic medical practice whose mission is to deliver comprehensive, compassionate medical care utilizing the combined talents of a team of dedicated, experienced, and extremely knowledgeable health care professionals each of whom is capable of approaching health-related issues from a unique point along the alternative care spectrum.

Ohio

Mansfield
Penhos, MD, Juan
Get Well Center

Address: 635 South Trimble Road
Mansfield, OH 44906

Phone: 419-524-2676
Fax: 419-524-2692
E-mail: juanpenhos@yahoo.com

Training Date: Trained with Dr. Ayre in 2007.
Conditions treated with IPT: Dr. Penhos treats cancer with IPT.
Practice Focus: Integrative medicine for cancer and other conditions.

Texas

Dallas/Ft. Worth (Grapevine)
Constantine A. Kotsanis, MD
The Kotsanis Institute

Address: 2020 W. Highway 114, Ste 260
Grapevine, TX 76051

Phone: 817-481-6342
Web site: www.kotsanisinstitute.com
E-mail: DrK@Kotsanisinstitute.com, info@kotsanisinstitute.com

Training Date: Trained with Dr. Perez Garcia in 2001.
Conditions treated with IPT: Dr. Kotsanis treats cancer with IPT.

Practice Focus: Treating the patient based on the individuals physical, metabolic, and biochemical makeup. He combines nutrition counseling, anti-aging therapies for different ailments. Dr. K. has been a practicing physician for twenty-five years. He conducts research, treats and educates physicians and patients alike. His mission is to change the way health is delivered to the world *one person at a time.*

License/Certifications
Dr. Kotsanis graduated from the University of Athens Medical School and completed residency in Otolaryngology from Loyola University of Chicago in 1983. He is Board Certified in Otolaryngology-Head and Neck Surgery, a fellow of the American Academy of Otolaryngic Allergy, and licensed by the Arizona State Board of Homeopathic

Medicine. A certified Clinical Nutritionist, he is also certified in Auditory Enhancement Therapy, IPT and is a certified IPT Instructor.

Wichita Falls
Jennings, MD, Lynn
The Champions Clinic

Address: 2934 Kemp Blvd.
Wichita Falls, TX 76308

Phone: 940-322-2400
Fax: 940-322-1930
Web site: www.thechampionsclinic.com
E-mail: fallsdoc@yahoo.com

Training Date: Trained with Dr. Perez Garcia in 2007.
Conditions treated with IPT: Dr. Jennings treats cancer with IPT.
Practice Focus: The clinic has chiropractors, doctors, and physical therapists on staff to restore normal biochemical health.

Washington

Clinton (Seattle)
Weeks, MD, Brad
The Weeks Clinic for Corrective Medicine and Psychiatry

Address: 6456 S. Central Ave PO Box 740
Clinton, WA 98236

Phone: 360-341-2303
Fax: 360-341-2313
Web site: http://weeksmd.com/
E-mail: admin@weeksmd.com

Training Date: Dr. Weeks trained with Dr. Ayre in 2002.
Conditions Treated with IPT: Cancer
Practice Focus: Dr. Weeks does not treat cancer. Instead, Dr. Weeks treats people (many of whom happen to have too many uncontrolled cancer cells).

Why is this distinction important? It is important because cancer is the illness that is most powerfully influenced by what the individual brings to the table: her or his will forces, spirit, and, most importantly, her or his reason for living.

Venezuela

Maracay
Martinez Leon, MD, PhD, Alberto
Consultorio Santa Maria

Address: Maracay, Venezuela

Phone: 243-554-7871
Fax: 243-554-7871 (same as Phone)
Web site: http://www.consultoriosantamaria.com.ve
E-mail: consultoriosantamaria@hotmail.com

Training Date: Trained with Dr. Perez Garcia in 2002.
Conditions treated with IPT: Dr. Martinez uses IPT to treat cancer and other conditions.
Practice Focus: In addition to being a certified IPT Instructor, Dr. Martinez also integrates ozone therapy and hyperbaric oxygen therapy in to his practice of treating cancer and other diseases.

ꔷ

APPENDIX C

Resources: Web Sites, Books and Articles

Books

The Official IPT/IPTLD™ Directory—www.IPTforcancer.com and **www. IPTLD.com** This site lists more information regarding IPTLD™ and allows you to find a practitioner.

Historical Information on IPTLD™—www.iptq.com Read more about IPTLD™ on the sites above or on the historical IPTLD™ Web site IPTQ. com

Researched Nutritionals—www.researchednutritionals.com
Our thanks to Researched Nutritionals for their ongoing support.

The Most Experienced IPTLD™ Doctor—www.donatoperezgarcia. com
Dr. Donato Perez Garcia III, grandson of the originator of IPTLD™ Chemotherapy. In 2007, Dr Garcia granted exclusivity of his training and speaking engagements regarding IPT/IPTLD™ to The Best Answer for Cancer FoundationSM. Dr. Garcia serves as the Senior Medical Advisor for the IOIP and the Foundation.

The U.S. Leader and Pioneer—www.contemporarymedicine.net
Dr. Steven Ayre, of Contemporary Medicine near Chicago/Midway Illinois, shares his years of IPTLD™ Chemotherapy learning with us. Dr. Ayre serves on The Best Answer for Cancer Foundation Board of Directors.

IPTLD™ Chemotherapy in Oceanside, California www.lesbreitmanmd.com After forty years of medical practice and seven years of practicing IPTLD™, Dr. Les Breitman feels so strongly about the efficacy of IPTLD™ Chemotherapy that he has made it the focal point of his medical practice. Dr. Breitman serves on The Best Answer for Cancer FoundationSM Board of Directors.

Clinical Trial of IPTLD™—www.elkabest.org/uruguay Since being published in December 2003, Eduardo Lasalvia-Prisca and his team have been researching on IPTLD™. Read the 2004 peer-reviewed publication of the clinical trial.

Beating Cancer Gently—www.beating-cancer-gently.com Compiled by Bill Henderson—a wealth of information and resources on compassionate cancer care, both complementary, alternate, and adjuvant.

Cancer: Treating Cancer with Insulin Potentiation Therapy
Learn how insulin can help target chemotherapy and be used as part of a comprehensive natural medicine approach to reverse cancer and cancer physiology. Ross A. Hauser, MD, Marion A. Hauser, MS, RD.

Cellular Cancer Therapy Through Modification of Blood Physico-Chemical Constants (Donation Therapy)
Donato Perez Garcia, MD (Donato 1) and Donato Perez Garcia y Bellon, MD (Donato 2) © 1978. Translation by Mike Dillinger.

Medicine of Hope, Insulin Cellular Therapy—www.IPTQ.org
The full text online in English and Spanish. This book provides an early history of IPT, how it works, numerous patient case studies and outcomes. Jean-Claude Paquette MD, © 1995. Translated from French by Aime' Ricci.

Cancer as a Turning Point: A Handbook for Cancer patients, Their Families and Health Professionals; You Can Fight For Your Life: Emotional Factors in the Treatment of Cancer; and How to Meditate: A Guide to Self-Discovery—www.cancerasaturningpoint.org

This book helps those dealing with cancer to find a "turning point" or spiritual understanding that can be used to promote healing and to find the unrealized dream within that can provide inspiration. Lawrence LeShan, PhD.

You Can Fight for Your Life: Emotional Factors in the Treatment of Cancer by Lawrence LeShan, Ph.D.
This work argues that the reason why clinical science has not solved the riddle of cancer may be that cancer might not lie totally within the realm of the laboratory. This work argues that the treatment of cancer may lie more in the mind and the emotions than in the body. It offers new evidence and insights into why some individuals get cancer ...

DVD—Reflections on the Lord's Prayer for People with Cancer—www.videovision.com
Ken Curtis explores coping with advanced cancer from personal experience based on the inspiration of the Twenty-Third Psalm.

Pure Soapbox—a cleansing jolt of perspective, motivation, and humor —www.e-junkie.com/ecom This book cannot get to you soon enough! Kimberlie Dykeman's fresh take on the power we all have inside is amazing. It's witty, funny, and downright brutal.

Web sites

The Best Answer for Cancer FoundationSM—The Best Answer for Cancer FoundationSM funds education and research to provide kinder, gentler chemotherapy—www.ElkaBest.org
The International Organization of IPT Physicians—www.IOIPcenter.org
The IOIP was established to coordinate the efforts and communication of the over three hundred trained IPTLD™ providers worldwide.

The IPTLD™ Patient/Survivor Center—www.IPTforcancer.com/center
This online discussion forum it free to all IPT/IPTLD™ patients, survivors, and concerned family/support personnel. The forum gives the patient the opportunity to visit with other patients and share their experiences or get answers to questions.

National Patient Travel Center—www.patienttravel.org The purpose of the National Patient Travel Center is "...to ensure that no financially needy patient is denied access to distant specialized medical evaluation, diagnosis, or treatment for lack of a means of long-distance medical air transportation."

Angel Flight—www.angelflight.com
Angel Flight primarily serves patients needing transportation to or from the heartland region.

Center for Advancement in Cancer Education (CACE)

Organization's Web site Mission: The Center for Advancement in Cancer Education (CACE) is a not-for-profit cancer education, counseling and referral agency providing nutritional, immunological and psychological resources for cancer prevention, prevention of recurrence, and support during and after treatment. Founded in 1977, the Center focuses on combining the body's natural healing potential with advances in medical science. The Center has provided prevention educational initiatives to thousands of laypersons and treatment support services to over thirty thousand patients, families, and health care professionals. caceinfo@comcast.net, 610-642-4810 http://shop.1asecure.com/index.cfm?StID=3661-6339, http://www.beatcancerkit.com/

Articles

The effect of insulin on chemotherapeutic drug sensitivity in human esophageal and lung cancer cells—www.ncbi.nlm.nih.gov/pubmed/12812659
Department of Oncology, General Hospital of People's Liberation Army Beijing 100853, China
Pretreatment with insulin enhances anticancer functions of 5-fluorouracil in human esophageal and colonic cancer cells—www.ncbi.nlm.nih.gov/pubmed/17439729
Institute of Biochemistry and Cell Biology, Shanghai Institutes for Biological Sciences, Chinese Academy of Sciences, Shanghai 200031, China.

Insulin for Cancer—www.time.com/time/magazine/article/0,09171,751277,00html
TIME Magazine, Monday, Mar. 09, 1925.

IPT: A New Concept in the Management of Chronic Degenerative Disease —www.iptforcancer.com
S. G. Ayre, D. Perez Garcia y Bellon and D. Perez Garcia, Jr.

IPT and Cachexia: A Dual-Purpose Approach to Cancer Management—www.iptforcancer.com
Ayre and Tisdale

New Approaches to the Delivery of Drugs to the Brain—www.iptforcancer.com
S.G. Ayre

Blood Brain-Barrier—www.iptforcancer.com
Ayre, Skaletski, and Mosnaim

Neoadjuvant Low-Dose Chemotherapy with Insulin in Breast Carcinomas—www.iptforcancer.com
S. G. Ayre, D. Perez Garcia y Bellon, and D. Perez Garcia, Jr.

Insulin, Chemotherapy and the Mechanisms of Malignancy: The Design and the Demise of Cancer—www.iptforcancer.com
S. G. Ayre, D. Perez Garcia y Bellon, and D. Perez Garcia, Jr.

Long-term effect of diabetes and its treatment on cognitive function—www.iptforcancer.com
New England Journal of Medicine

Insulin-induced enhancement of antitumoral response to methotrexate in breast cancer patients—www.iptforcancer.com
Uruguay Study

The risk of developing uterine sarcoma after tamoxifen use—www.blackwell-synergy.com/doi/abs/
International Journal of Gynecological Cancer

The Insulin Potentiation Therapy(Ipt) in The Treatment of Chronical and Oncological Diseases—www.infoforcancer.com
Journal MED

APPENDIX D

History of IPT/IPTLD™

The Inception of Insulin Potentiation Targeted LowDose™ Therapy

Insulin Potentiation Targeted LowDose™ (IPTLD™)* was initially developed in 1930 for the treatment of human disease by Donato Perez Garcia I. MD (1896-1971). A surgeon lieutenant in the Mexican military establishment, his preliminary work with insulin involved an innovative course of self-treatment for a gastrointestinal problem that he suffered from for years. All previous treatments had failed to resolve it.

When he first learned of the then newly discovered hormone insulin being used to treat diabetes, he noted that, in addition to diabetes, its use was also indicated for the treatment of nondiabetic malnutrition. So he decided to try it on himself. The treatment was completely successful; his symptoms disappeared and his weight became normal.

Reflecting on his own experience, Dr. Perez Garcia did what many innovators in the medical field do: he asked himself why. He considered that the insulin might have helped his body tissues assimilate the food he had eaten and wondered if perhaps insulin might help tissues assimilate medications.

This led to the unique technique that Drs. Donato Perez Garcia, Jr., MD, his son Donato Perez Garcia III, MD ,and Steven G. Ayre, MD, eventually developed to treat cancer. **The technique became known as Insulin Potentiation Therapy (IPT).** [Insulin Potentiation Targeted LowDose™ (IPTLD™) is the current name (researched, reserved and assigned in 2006 by Annie Brandt of The Best Answer for Cancer FoundationSM to more accurately describe the therapy) for that same procedure. Only the name has changed; the procedure is the same. The names are used interchangeably throughout this book and should be considered synonymous. When reporting historical events, we will use the historical name IPT.]

While IPTLD™ can be used to treat and manage a variety of diseases, its application in cancer management is particularly ingenious. These physicians recognized the possibility that giving cancer cells insulin would prime cell membranes to open up. Coordinating this event with the introduction of low-dose chemotherapy, it is believed that much more of the chemotherapy drugs are able to get inside the cancer cells to kill them. At the same time, healthy cells are left unharmed. This process allows patients to avoid the worst of the dangerous and undesirable side effects caused by traditional, higher-dosage chemotherapy treatments.

First Clinical Use of IPT

Dr. Perez Garcia first performed IPT on a patient in 1930. Carlos Sosa had neurosyphilis, an illness that affects the brain and was, at the time, considered incurable. Using salts of mercury and arsenic (standard treatment for syphilis then) in combination with insulin, Dr. Perez Garcia achieved a radical cure for Mr. Sosa (penicillin and other antibiotics that would eventually be used to treat syphilis did not appear until after 1940). In the newspaper *El Universal* (January 14, 1930), Mr. Sosa told a reporter about his suffering and his remarkable recuperation. He lived until the late 1970s.

The World Takes Notice

In 1937, Dr. Perez Garcia was invited to the United States to demonstrate his therapy at the Austin State Hospital in Austin, Texas, and at St. Elizabeth's Hospital in Washington, D.C. Upon his return to Mexico, Dr. Perez Garcia managed a military medical clinic where he produced powerful clinical results in significant numbers of his patients with applications of his IPT therapy.

In 1943, the doctor was invited to treat some patients at the San Diego Naval Hospital, where he effected more of the same positive changes in patients suffering from neurosyphilis, malaria, rheumatic fever, and cholecystitis. The results led to a write-up of Dr. Perez Garcia and his "insulin treatments" in the April 10, 1944, edition of *TIME* magazine, titled "Insulin for Everything."

Trio of Medical Doctors Develop IPT in the Scientific Medical Community

Donato Perez Garcia, Jr., MD, and his son Donato Perez Garcia III, MD, followed in the developer's footsteps, both learning and practicing IPT in Mexico. A third doctor, Steven G. Ayre, MD, became caught up in the enthusiasm and promise surrounding this treatment technique and visited the Mexico City clinic of Dr. Donato Perez Garcia, Jr., in the summer of 1976 to receive training in IPT. Since that summer, Dr. Ayre has worked closely with the Drs. Donato Perez Garcia over the following decades to develop IPT through trials and research, writing five peer-reviewed scientific journal articles and making several presentations in an effort to develop IPT through many studies and trials.

One such presentation occurred in 1996 when Drs. Donato Perez Garcia, Jr., and Steven G. Ayre presented IPT at the Forty-Second Annual Symposium on Fundamental Cancer Research held at the prestigious MD Anderson Institute in Houston, Texas. In response to the winds of change, the institute set up its own Center for Alternative Medicine Research. Motivated by the compelling clinical evidence presented at this 1996 symposium, investigators associated with that institution undertook a firsthand look at the "Mexican – Insulin Potentiation Therapy." After reviewing the clinical evidence gathered through Dr. Donato Garcia Perez Jr's clinic in Mexico City and Dr. Donato Garcia Perez III's clinic in Tijuana, the investigator who performed the site visits at both clinics remarked, "This is incredible. How come nothing has ever been done about this before?"

Due to the concerted efforts of people at the MD Anderson Institute, an invitation was extended to the trio of IPT doctors to present the scientific background on IPT, including some case presentations from the clinical work done in Mexico. This presentation was made at the National Institutes of Health, Office of Alternative Medicine POMES conference in August of 1997.

Another invitation was extended to Drs. Perez Garcia, Jr., and Ayre to make a Best Case Series presentation before the members of the Cancer Advisory Panel of the Office of Complementary and Alternative Medicine at the National Institutes of Health in Bethesda, Maryland. Drs. Ayre and Perez Garcia, Jr., made this presentation on September 18, 2000. The panel members were impressed with the cases presented; however, it was claimed that there was insufficient data to warrant any action to formally study IPT at that time. The IPT physicians were counseled to produce more prospective treatment data and to make another Best Case Series presentation in the future. This work is now under way.

The Status of IPTLD™ Today

During the eighty-year development of Insulin Potentiation Therapy, those who have administered it and documented its use have held the conviction that the therapy is valuable, and that knowledge of it should be made widely available to the medical profession. But, as IPTLD™'s proponents have learned, "you can't push the river." It became clear to them that the way to accomplish their goals is to work quietly and diligently, treating those patients who ask for help, documenting all results, publishing these results in medical journals, and develop, as funding permits, more sophisticated clinical trials. The Drs. Perez Garcia and Dr. Ayre have learned that "the river will flow, ceaselessly, at its own pace." But they take comfort in knowing that the river is always changing course.

*The name IPT (Insulin Potentiation Therapy has recently been changed to IPTLD™ (Insulin Potentiation Targeted LowDose™). **IPTLD™** is the current name (researched, reserved and assigned in 2006 by Annie Brandt and the Board of The Elka Best Foundation to more accurately describe the therapy) for that same procedure. Only the name has changed; the therapy remains the same. Throughout this book, you will see both names. Please consider them synonymous.*

APPENDIX E

IPTLD™ Treatment at a Glance

The IPTLD™ Advantage: Tougher on Cancer. Easier on Patients.

Insulin Potentiation Targeted Therapy Low Dose™ (IPTLD™) is a relatively new (first used on cancer in 1946, but only recently discovered by the world), proven (through the years and the tens of thousands of cancer patients), and powerful approach to treating cancer. It utilizes traditional FDA-approved chemotherapeutic drugs **in fractionated doses** and insulin to more effectively transport the drugs across cell membranes into the cancer cells instead of the healthy cells.

IPTLD™ vs. Traditional Chemotherapy Treatment

One outstanding advantage IPTLD™ has over traditional treatment is that a much lower dose of chemotherapeutic drugs is required. IPTLD™ **selectively targets cancer cells** while affecting relatively few normal cells. Therefore, patients do not suffer the severe side effects that commonly occur with conventional chemotherapy, such as hair loss, vomiting, fatigue, and depression. In addition, there is no damage to the patient's immune system or vital body organs. Thus, the quality of a patient's life is significantly improved in comparison to that many patients experience when undergoing conventional treatment experience.

A Closer Look at How it Works

Cancer cells derive energy from an unlimited supply of glucose, which they get by secreting their own insulin. They also stimulate their own growth by producing insulin-like growth factors (IGF). These are the mechanisms of malignancy.

Insulin and IGF each work by attaching to specific cell membrane receptors, which are much more concentrated on cancer cell membranes than on normal ones. Attachment to these receptors is key to the success of IPTLD™ and helps explain why it is able to use lower doses of drugs that mainly target the cancer cells, kill them more effectively, and avoid the dose-related side effects of traditional chemotherapy.

In effect, IPTLD™ kills cancer cells by using the same mechanisms that cancer cells use to kill people.

A One-Two Punch

Insulin, in addition to its ability to help deliver higher levels of the chemotherapy drugs into the cancer cells, also causes these cells to go into their growth phase where they actually become more vulnerable to the chemotherapy drugs. The cells are hit harder and at a time when they are most vulnerable to the assault, thus maximizing results.

In 1981, a study conducted at George Washington University showed that the chemotherapy drug, methotrexate, when used with insulin, increased the drug's cell-killing effect by a factor of 10,000!

This study was done in conjunction with the Laboratory of Pathophysiology at NCI, which studied the impact of methotrexate on breast cancer with and without insulin. The study concluded that 10-10 methotrexate without insulin was equivalent to 10-6 when combined with insulin. This 1981 study found a specific enhancement of a particular carrier system for methotrexate, but launched additional interest in studying IPTLD™ and its broader applications. Additional research found that because insulin recruits resting cancer cells to become active in protein and DNA synthesis, they become more vulnerable to the targeted activity of chemotherapy. As an added advantage, insulin assists debilitated cancer patients with appetite and metabolism, helping to resolve the wasting that accompanies the disease and its therapy. (Source: Alabaster, O. Metabolic modification by insulin enhances methotrexate cytotoxicity in MCF-7 human breast cancer. Europe J Cancer Oncol. 1981; 17:1223-1228.)

IPTLD™ Facilitates Comprehensive Cancer Care

Effectively fighting cancer is hard work that involves more than medical treatment alone. It requires a comprehensive approach.

Because IPTLD™ spares its recipients from the debilitating side effects experienced with conventional treatment, patients are more able and more motivated to pursue the work necessary for their own well-being. Conventional chemotherapy treatment can be so taxing that patients won't even consider, let alone take action on, other cancer-fighting measures such as diet modification, exercise, detox programs, and mind-body medicine.

What it is Like to Receive IPTLD™

The patient arrives at the clinic in a fasting state, and an IV of saline solution is inserted into a vein in the arm. Their vital stats are then taken, including their fasting blood sugar level. A dose of insulin based on their body weight is injected into the IV line. The patient is then closely monitored for symptoms of hypoglycemia, or low blood sugar. After about twenty-five minutes, or once symptoms appear, the blood sugar level is taken again. Patients will feel very hungry, and it would not be unusual to experience mild and temporary symptoms of hypoglycemia, which can include fatigue, headache, or sweating.

When it is determined that the blood sugar level is in a certain range, this is called the therapeutic moment and it is at this point that the chemo drugs are administered through the IV. Immediately following these drugs, a dose of glucose is administered, and the treatment is finished. From start to finish, the treatment usually takes anywhere from one to two hours. Because there are little or no side effects, the patient can usually go on with his or her regular daily events.

Again, IPTLD™ is exciting because it allows so many of its patients to devote full attention to their wellness, thus increasing their chances of recovery, and improving the quality and duration of their lives.

❦

APPENDIX F

Glossary*

Adrenal cortical level – The level of cortisone (a hormone produced by the adrenal cortex) found in the adrenal gland or tissue.

Alternative Medicine – Alternative medicine is commonly categorized together with <u>complementary medicine</u> under the umbrella term "<u>complementary and alternative medicine</u>" (<u>CAM</u>). Alternative medicine has been described as "any of various systems of healing or treating disease (as <u>chiropractic</u>, <u>homeopathy</u>, or <u>faith healing</u>) not included in the traditional <u>medical</u> curricula taught in the United States and Britain."

Amygdala – One of two small, almond-shaped masses of gray matter that are part of the limbic system and are located in the temporal lobes of the cerebral hemispheres. Also called *amygdaloid nucleus*.

Anaerobic organisms – Organisms that have the ability to sustain life in an atmosphere devoid of oxygen

ANS – Autonomic Nervous System – The portion of the nervous system concerned with regulation of activity of cardiac muscle, smooth muscle, and glands, usually restricted to the sympathetic and parasympathetic nervous systems.

Antimicrobial – Tending to destroy microbes, prevent their development, or inhibit their pathogenic action.

Antiviral – Destroying or inhibiting the growth and reproduction of viruses.

ATP – Units of energy. Adenosine triphosphate; an adenosine-derived nucleotide that supplies large amounts of energy to cells for various biochemical processes, including muscle contraction and sugar metabolism, through its hydrolysis to ADP.

Ascorbates – A compound or derivative of ascorbic acid (vitamin C).

Autologous stem cells – Cells derived or transferred from the same individual's body: *autologous blood donation; an autologous bone marrow transplant.*

Avastin – Bevacizumab (trade name Avastin) is a <u>monoclonal antibody</u> against <u>vascular endothelial growth factor</u>. It is used in the treatment of <u>cancer</u>, where it inhibits tumor growth by blocking <u>the formation of new blood vessels</u>. Bevacizumab was the first clinically available <u>angiogenesis inhibitor</u> in the United States.

Biofeedback – Biofeedback is a form of <u>alternative medicine</u> that involves measuring a subject's bodily processes such as <u>blood pressure</u>, <u>heart rate</u>, skin temperature, <u>galvanic skin response</u> (<u>sweating</u>), and muscle tension and conveying such information to him or her in real time in order to raise his or her <u>awareness</u> and conscious control of the related physiological activities. By providing access to <u>physiological</u> information about which the user is generally unaware, biofeedback allows users to gain control over physical processes previously considered <u>automatic</u>.

Cancer – Cancer is a group of <u>diseases</u> in which <u>cells</u> are *aggressive* (grow and <u>divide</u> without respect to normal limits), *invasive* (invade and destroy adjacent tissues), and/or *metastatic* (spread to other locations in the body). These three <u>malignant</u> properties of cancers differentiate them from <u>benign tumors</u>, which are self-limited in their growth and do not invade or metastasize (although some benign tumor types are capable of becoming malignant).

Carcinogenic – The term carcinogen refers to any substance, <u>radionuclide</u>, or radiation that is an agent directly involved in the promotion of <u>cancer</u> or in the facilitation of its propagation. This may be due to <u>genomic instability</u> or to the disruption of cellular <u>metabolic</u> processes. Several radioactive substances are considered carcinogens, but their carcinogenic activity is attributed to the radiation, for example gamma rays or alpha particles, which they emit. Common examples of carcinogens are inhaled asbestos and tobacco smoke.

Cholecystitis – is inflammation of the gallbladder.

Ciliary body of the iris – The ciliary body is the circumferential tissue inside the eye composed of the ciliary muscle and ciliary processes. It is part of the uveal tract—the layer of tissue which provides most of the nutrients in the eye. There are three sets of ciliary muscles in the eye, the longitudinal, radial, and circular muscles. They are near the front of the eye, above and below the lens. They are attached to the lens by connective tissue called the zonule of Zinn, and are responsible for shaping the lens to focus light on the retina.

Complementary medicine – Complementary medicine refers to a group of therapeutic and diagnostic disciplines that exist largely outside the institutions where conventional health care is taught and provided.[1] As its name suggests, complementary medicine differs from alternative medicine in that it does not offer a competing (or 'alternative') viewpoint to that based on science-based knowledge. Even so, the two are commonly categorized together as complementary and alternative medicine (CAM).

Concomitant – Accompanying, accessory, joined with another.

Cortical Releasing Factor – CRF – *n* substance secreted by the hypothalamus that triggers the pituitary-adrenal axis. The increased release of this substance plays a significant role in immunosuppression and has other secondary effects. Also called *CRF*. Corticotropin-releasing factor.

Cortisone – A naturally occurring corticosteroid that functions primarily in carbohydrate metabolism and is used in the treatment of rheumatoid arthritis, adrenal insufficiency, certain allergies, and gout.

CT Scan – An image produced by computer tomography.

Cytokine production by white blood cells – A generic term for nonantibody proteins released by one cell population on contact with specific antigen, which act as intercellular mediators, as in the generation of an immune response.

Cytotoxic effect – having a deleterious effect upon cells.

Debridement – The process of removing nonliving tissue from pressure ulcers, <u>burns</u>, and other <u>wounds</u>. Wounds that contain non-living (necrotic) tissue take longer to heal. The necrotic tissue may become colonized with bacteria, producing an unpleasant odor. Though the wound is not necessarily infected, the bacteria can cause inflammation and strain the body's ability to fight infection. Necrotic tissue may also hide pockets of pus called abscesses.

Deep relaxation/meditation/visualization – These tools promote emotional and physical peace, which stimulates your immune system to function optimally for the benefit of your health.

Detoxification – Detoxification is one of the more widely used treatments and concepts in alternative medicine. It is based on the principle that illnesses can be caused by the accumulation of toxic substances (toxins) in the body. Eliminating existing toxins and avoiding new toxins are essential parts of the healing process. Detoxification utilizes a variety of tests and techniques.

EFT—Emotional Freedom Technique – This is a simple acupressure technique that anyone can learn. It dramatically and quickly dissolves negative emotions that can be very harmful to your health.

Emotion Code – This is a muscle testing technique to identify and release personal and inherited trapped emotions.

Epigenetic phenomena – Pertaining to <u>epigenesis</u>. Altering the activity of <u>genes</u> without changing their structure. Something seen a sign that is often associated with a specific illness or condition and is therefore diagnostically important.

Forgiveness Work – Many people say to "forgive and forget." But, how do you forgive? Using the lessons of Byron Katie, acupressure, spirituality, and Radical Forgiveness, she will guide you to "let go" of that unhealthy baggage that can slow down your healing.

Glycolysis – Primitive energy production. The anaerobic enzymatic conversion of glucose to the simpler compounds lactate or pyruvate, resulting in energy stored in the form of ATP, as occurs in muscle.

Hippocampus – Part of the limbic system. A curved elevation in the floor of the inferior horn of the lateral ventricle; a functional component of the limbic system, its efferent projections form the fornix of the hippocampus.

Hypertension – Hypertension is high blood pressure. Blood pressure is the force of blood pushing against the walls of arteries as it flows through them. Arteries are the blood vessels that carry oxygenated blood from the heart to the body's tissues.

Hypoglycemic – pertaining to or resembling a state of low blood glucose level.

Hypothyroidism – Underactive thyroid.

Ig A levels – Abbreviation for Immunoglobulin A. Immune globulin – a class of proteins produced in lymph tissue in vertebrates and that function as antibodies in the immune response.

Insulin – A polypeptide hormone secreted by the islets of Langerhans and functioning in the regulation of the metabolism of carbohydrates and fats, especially the conversion of glucose to glycogen, which lowers the blood glucose level.

Integrative Medicine – Integrative medicine is a branch of alternative medicine which claims to limit itself to methods with strong scientific evidence of efficacy and safety. The main proponent of integrative medicine is Andrew T. Weil, MD, who founded the Program in Integrative Medicine at the University of Arizona in 1994 based on a phrase coined by Elson Haas, MD.

Interleukin – Any of a class of cytokines that act to stimulate, regulate, or modulate lymphocytes such as T cells. *Interleukin-1*, which has two subtypes, is released by macrophages and certain other cells, and regulates cell-mediated and humoral immunity. It induces the production of interleukin-2 by helper T cells and also acts as a pyrogen.

Interleukin-2 stimulates the proliferation of helper T cells, stimulates B cell growth and differentiation, and has been used experimentally to treat cancer. *Interleukin-3* is released by mast cells and helper T cells in response to an antigen and stimulates the growth of blood stem cells and lymphoid cells such as macrophages and mast cells. There are many other interleukins that are part of the immune system.

In vitro – In an artificial environment outside the living organism.

IPT – Insulin Potentiation Therapy – Insulin potentiation therapy ("IPT") is an <u>alternative medicine</u> therapy that uses <u>Food and Drug Administration</u>-approved <u>cancer</u>-fighting drugs in lower doses. It is used by some alternative medicine practitioners to treat cancer and other diseases because the lower dosing of drug eliminates many of the debilitating side effects of conventional <u>chemotherapy</u>. This treatment is also sometimes referred to as "low-dose chemotherapy."

IPTLD™ – Insulin Potentiation Targeted LowDose™ therapy is a targeted low-dose form of chemotherapy.

Kinases -Kinase – an enzyme that catalyzes the conversion of a proenzyme to an active enzyme <u>enzyme</u> – any of several complex proteins that are produced by cells and act as catalysts in specific biochemical reactions

Krebs cycle – A series of enzymatic reactions in aerobic organisms involving oxidative metabolism of acetyl units and producing high-energy phosphate compounds, which serve as the main source of cellular energy. Also called *citric acid cycle, tricarboxylic acid cycle.*

Limbic system – A group of interconnected structures of the brain including the hypothalamus, amygdala, and hippocampus that are located beneath the cortex, are common to all mammals, and are associated with emotions such as fear and pleasure, memory, motivation, and various autonomic functions.

Macrophages – Any of the large phagocytic cells of the reticuloendothelial system. Phagocyte – a cell or protozoan that engulfs particles, such as microorganisms [Greek *phagein* to eat + *kutos* vessel].

Malaria – An infectious disease characterized by cycles of chills, fever, and sweating, caused by a protozoan of the genus *Plasmodium* in red blood cells, which is transmitted to humans by the bite of an infected female anopheles mosquito.

Mind-Body Medicine – is the practice of medicine based upon the scientific understanding of the biochemical underpinnings of awareness and consciousness. it is the practice of medicine with an understanding that the "mind and the body are one, and that our emotions and feelings are the bridge that links the two.

Misoneism – The fear of change or innovation and the hatred of new things.

Modalities – *Medicine* A therapeutic method or agent, such as surgery, chemotherapy, or electrotherapy, that involves the physical treatment of a disorder.

Necrotic – Death of cells or tissues through injury or disease, especially in a localized area of the body.

Neurohormones – A hormone secreted by or acting on a part of the nervous system.

Neurotransmitters – A chemical substance, such as acetylcholine or dopamine, that transmits nerve impulses across a synapse.

PET Scan – Short for *positron emission tomography scan*. A cross-sectional image of a metabolic process in a human or animal body produced by positron emission tomography.

Potentiate – To make stronger. Increase the effect of or act synergistically with a drug or a physiological or biochemical phenomenon.

Pseudomonas infection – type genus of the family Pseudomonadaceae, <u>bacteria genus</u> – a genus of bacteria. A bacterial infection.

Psychoneuroimmunology – (PNI) is the study of the interaction between psychological processes and the nervous and immune systems of the human body.[1] PNI has an interdisciplinary approach, interlacing disciplines as psychology, neuroscience, immunology, physiology, pharmacology, psychiatry, behavioral medicine, infectious diseases, endocrinology, rheumatology and others.

The main interest of PNI is the interaction between the nervous and immune systems, and the relation between mind processes and health. PNI studies, among other things, the physiological functioning of the neuroimmune system in health and disease; disorders of the neuroimmune system (autoimmune diseases, hypersensitivities, immune deficiency), the physical, chemical, and physiological characteristics of the components of the neuroimmune system in vitro, in situ, and in vivo.

Rheumatic fever – Rheumatic fever is an inflammatory disease that may develop after a Group A streptococcal infection (such as strep throat or scarlet fever) and can involve the heart, joints, skin, and brain.

Salvarsan – The arsenic containing agent used to treat syphilis.

Spiritual Growth – Creating peace, love, and joy in your life. Understanding the purpose of life. Gratitude and prayer work.

Sympathetic nervous system – The sympathetic nervous system (SNS) is a branch of the autonomic nervous system. It is always active at a basal level (called sympathetic tone) and becomes more active during times of stress. Its actions during the stress response comprise the fight-or-flight response.

T3, T4 Thyroid hormones – The thyroid hormones, thyroxine (T_4) and triiodothyronine (T_3), are tyrosine-based hormones produced by the thyroid gland. An important component in the synthesis is iodine. The major form of thyroid hormone in the blood is thyroxine (T_4). The ratio of T_4 to T_3 released in the blood is roughly 20 to 1. Thyroxine is converted to the active T_3 (three to four times more potent than T_4) within cells by deiodinases (5'-iodinase). These are further processed by decarboxylation and deiodination to produce iodothyronamine (T_1a) and thyronamine (T_0a).

Most of the thyroid hormone circulating in the <u>blood</u> is bound to transport <u>proteins</u>. Only a very small fraction of the circulating hormone is free (unbound) and biologically active, hence measuring concentrations of free thyroid hormones is of great diagnostic value.

TSH – Thyroid-stimulating hormone (also known as TSH or thyrotropin) is a hormone synthesized and secreted by <u>thyrotrope</u> cells in the <u>anterior pituitary gland</u> that regulates the endocrine function of the <u>thyroid gland.[1]</u>

"Therapeutic moment" – A point when all cancer cells have become saturated with insulin and are permeable (easy passage); while all of the non-cancerous cells in the body are only partially saturated with insulin and therefore, not completely permeable. This is the time when low dose (approximately 10% of standard) chemotherapeutic drugs are administered intravenously.

Thyroglobulin panel – a blood test used primarily to detect well-differentiated thyroid cancers.

Tertiary Neurosyphilis – The final stage of neurosyphilis, following a latent period that may last years, characterized by spread of the disease to many organs and tissues, including the skin, bones, joints, heart, brain, and spinal cord. Syphilis is an infectious systemic disease that may be either congenital or acquired through sexual contact or contaminated needles.

Type 2 diabetes – A metabolic disease characterized by abnormally high levels of glucose in the blood, caused by an acquired resistance to insulin. Type 2 diabetes appears during adulthood, usually in overweight or elderly individuals, and is treated with oral medication or insulin. People with either type of diabetes benefit from dietary restriction of sugars and other carbohydrates. Uncontrolled blood glucose levels increase the risk for long-term medical complications including peripheral nerve disease, retinal damage, kidney disease, and progressive atherosclerosis caused by damage to endothelial cells in blood vessels, leading to coronary artery disease and peripheral vascular disease.

Tumoricidal – Of or being destructive to tumor cells

*Source: **http://encyclopedia.thefreedictionary.com/canceres**

Note: Underlined words are hyperlinked to The Free Dictionary Web site.

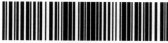

12243628R00090

Made in the USA
Charleston, SC
22 April 2012